Recent Advances in Pet Nutrition

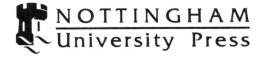

NOTTINGHAM
University Press

Nottingham University Press
Manor Farm, Main Street, Thrumpton
Nottingham, NG11 0AX, United Kingdom

NOTTINGHAM

First published 2006
© The several contributors names in the list of contents

British Library Cataloguing in Publication Data
Recent Advances in Pet Nutrition
I. Laue, D., II. Tucker, L.A.

ISBN 10: 1-904761-11-9
ISBN 13: 978-1-904761-11-2

Disclaimer

Every reasonable effort has been made to ensure that the material in this book is true,
correct, complete and appropriate at the time of writing. Nevertheless, the publishers and
authors do not accept responsibility for any omission or error, or for any injury, damage,
loss or financial consequences arising from the use of the book.

Typeset by Nottingham University Press, Nottingham
Printed and bound by Hobbs the Printers, Hampshire, England

CONTENTS

Introduction

In the last decade, pet nutritionists have found it increasingly difficult to keep up to date with developments in science relating to the field of pet nutrition. Despite this, great advances in the understanding of nutrition and its impact on health have been made over recent years.

The fields of gut development, gut microflora, immunology and the role of glycomics are all linked to pet health. Mycotoxin contamination of petfood is now an important media issue, and new disciplines, such as glycomics and nutrigenomics, have generated much interest in recent years. Human health trends are increasingly reflected in the petfood industry, with research projects now showing overlap between humans and pets.

To give nutritionists, veterinarians and petfood manufacturers a concise and focused review of the current and future state of pet nutrition, seminars have been held by the specialist feed ingredients company, Alltech, covering several species and topics. The key objective of the seminars was to examine current problems in petfood and how natural forms of technical feed ingredients may overcome them. Topics include the use of specialist yeast derivatives, natural forms of minerals, mycotoxin contamination and the use of antioxidants for increased food stability.

The "Recent Advances in Pet Nutrition" book owes its existence to the labour and commitment of many contributors to whom we are indeed grateful.

As part of an expanding series of specialist nutrition-focused seminars, the topics covered have generated great interest amongst many delegates from a spectrum of pet nutritionists and petfood manufacturers from different parts of the world.

We trust that readers of the papers will also find them as stimulating.

Dr. Doerte-Katja Laue
Dr Lucy Tucker

November 2006

A changing landscape: the pet food market in Europe

Juergen Zentek and Doerte-Katja Laue

The European pet food market has continuously expanded during recent decades. This is due to a long lasting growth in pet ownership, the decreasing use of table scraps and the general move towards convenience foods. In recent years, pet food trends in Western Europe have changed, and the growth rate of the market has slowed in many countries so that a mature market situation has developed. The market has split into several distinct segments, as pet owner's demands for premium products and sophisticated accessories for their animals have led to an increase in demand. At the other end of the scale, there remains an obvious requirement for pet foods that fulfil the nutritional needs of the animals at a reasonable price, a situation that has been strengthened by unfavourable economic situations in some countries.

Another important factor for consideration in the pet food markets is the current and future expansion of the European Union. Applicant countries offer promising opportunities due to lower level of calorie coverage in prepared pet food and the expected growth of pet ownership and pet food purchasing. Even in the established EU member states, considerable differences exist in pet food markets between countries. Even when the standard of living is more or less comparable, there are obvious differences in habits of keeping pets and the traditions of pet feeding that affect the market, as Europe is by no means uniform in its consumer choices. Differences include population density, proportion of dogs and cats, calorie coverage by commercial pet foods and the balance between commercial foods and traditional method of feeding pets, such as self cooked food and table scraps.

The European pet population in 2006

The numbers of households that contain pets are estimated to have reached 55 million by the European Pet Food Industry Federation (FEDIAF). The number of cats is higher compared to dogs, with

1

approximately 47 million cats and 41 million dogs kept in Western European countries (FEDIAF, 2004). A population of 35 million pet birds, 9 million aquaria and 36 million other species, which are mainly rodents and small mammals, but also include reptiles, should be considered an important and growing segment of the marketplace.

In the last decade, changes in pet ownership have been observed. Dog populations tend to be stable or (in some countries) slightly decreasing, whilst the number of cats is increasing. Based on the 155.6 million households in Western Europe, it can be estimated that 21% have dogs and 20% cats, with an average number of 1.1 dogs and 1.4 cats per household (FEDIAF, 2004). Spain has the greatest numbers of pet dogs out of all EU countries, with 13 million. They are followed by France, with 8.5 million, and Great Britain, with 6.9 million (Royal Canin / PET in Europe, 2006).

The number of cats has increased recently, as has the tendency to keep more than one cat per household, which is seen in many countries (ZZF, 2001). This reflects the popularity of cats as a 'lifestyle adapted' pet and may also be explained by recommendations to facilitate socialisation by keeping more than one cat, especially in households where cats are alone for long periods during the day and may resort to destructive behavioural patterns.

The trend towards fewer dogs is also due to changing lifestyles, where people have less time to devote to exercising them, for example. The selection of dogs as household pets has also been subject to other social influences. External factors have had great impact on public opinion towards dogs, highlighting the topic of responsible ownership. Discussions relating to the role of dogs in urban environments, regarding problems with public hygiene, and additional controversies following unfortunate accidents with 'dangerous' and 'aggressive' dogs have reduced the popularity of these animals.

Table 1 shows the changes in the German dog population, which is one of the five countries (together with France, the United Kingdom, Italy and Spain) in Western Europe exerting a strong economic impact on the pet food industry.

The stable or negative trend in the dog population is also observed with regard to breed and size preferences. In Europe, the number of small sized dogs (< 10 kg BW) was estimated to be 34%, with medium and large breeds comprising 37% and 29% of the total population respectively (Euromonitor, 2001). The increasing popularity of small dogs is global, due to their reduced exercise

Year	Number of puppies
2005	90306
2004	92602
2003	91227
2002	90257
2001	89822
2000	88659
1999	97860
1998	106815
1997	114670
1996	117893
1995	119460
1994	114690
1993	109785
1992	106490

Table 1. Number of puppies registered by the German Kennel Club (VDH, 2006)

requirements and smaller modern houses and increased apartment dwelling. Japan has a national passion for small breed canines, which form 78% of all whelpings. In countries outside Asia, e.g. Germany, USA and Brazil small breeds represent around 45% of births (Royal Canin / PETS International Magazine, 2006).

The age structure of canines in Western Europe is highly variable, with an estimated 9% being under two years old and 16% being more than 10 years old. The number of older animals in the United Kingdom (23%), the Netherlands (21%), France (18%), and Germany (17%) is above the European average, whereas fewer aged animals are seen in Portugal (7%), Norway (11%), Italy and Spain (12%) (Euromonitor, 2001).

In contrast to the dog population, the number of cats has increased steadily in recent years; a development that has huge economic consequences for the related industries. Opinions regarding the age of cat populations in Europe differ, but in most Western European countries the number of cats is considered to be either stable or increasing. France, the United Kingdom, Italy and Germany have the biggest cat populations (Euromonitor, 2001). Whilst the number of cats kept differs by country, the estimated average number of cats in Western Europe is 1.4 per household. Households with more than one cat are seen frequently in Austria (average 2.2 cats), Switzerland (1.8), Belgium (1.8), Norway (1.8), Spain (1.7), the United Kingdom (1.6), and Italy (1.6). Twenty-six percent of the total cat population is younger than two years and 18% is older than 10 years. Countries with a higher population of older cats include the United Kingdom (29%), the Netherlands (23%), Germany (22%), Sweden (21%), and Switzerland (19%).

The situation in the EU 'application' countries and in Eastern Europe is more difficult to clarify due to a scarcity of statistical data. Recent data indicates a dog population in Czech Republic of 0.9 million and a cat population of 0.7 million. Numbers for Slovakia reveal 0.6 million dogs and 0.3 million cats. (AC Nielsen / PETS International Magazine, 2005). There is an estimated pet population of 35.7 million in Russia, 14.6 million pets in Poland, 4.8 million pets in Czech Republic and 4.5 million pets in Hungary (ZZF, 2005).

Demographic and social factors

Several facts must be taken into consideration when speculating about the future of the European pet food market. The current human population dynamics in Europe show negative trends in many countries, with slowing birth rates, and a higher elderly population. In many countries there is a strong trend towards increased urbanisation and a higher number of households with fewer people per household. In addition, lifestyles have changed. Individualisation is important for many younger people, and the length of time a person is out of the house during the day or even for longer periods has increased.

Traditionally, population mobility has been less in the European Union compared to other parts of the world, but due to changes in economic conditions and lifestyles of young people, this has increased in recent years. Taking figures for Germany as an example (ZZF, 2001) most pets are kept by owners aged 35 – 49 years (39% of all pets) with a clear relationship seen between pet numbers and the number of family members. Pets are often kept in families with at least one child (46% of all pets), lower frequencies are found in single households (22%) and with couples without children (32%), according to statistical evaluation from 30,500 interviews (ZZF, 2003). According to these findings, couples without children and single people, represent, on a household basis, 60% of cat owners, 59% of dog owners, 58% of the pet bird owners and 48% of the aquarium owners. This fact is important, because it can be expected that the number of households of single people or couples without children, will increase in future, making up about 72% of the total number of households by 2010. If current trends continue, populations of cats and other more convenient companion animals will continue to increase in the future, as they are more suitable for this type of household structure and lifestyle than dogs.

Another recent trend is the market for small mammals and reptiles, which represents a growing segment in the pet food market. The popularity of these species is based on low-cost and maintenance, and the market for these types of pets grew by 32% between 1998 and 2004 (Euromonitor, PETS International Magazine, 2005).

Such demographic trends are comparable in many other EU member states, as changing lifestyles of pet owners affect the development of pet markets. More importantly, these changes can also influence the position of the companion animal in society. Humanisation of pets is obvious, and can be explained by pets establishing specific roles as social partners. This development has been taken on board and is now actively supported by the marketing strategies of pet food and supplier companies. Seeing pets as beings with similar or equal requirements as their human owners opens up new marketing opportunities, as people wish to spend more money on indulging their animals.

Pet food industry and market expectations

The market for pet food and its related products is now mature in most Western European countries. Volumes of dog food are on the wane in several countries, inducing a general fall of pet food volumes, but not necessarily in revenues generated from those sales. FEDIAF (2004) puts the total number of pet food companies in Europe at 450, and the current production volume of all pet food is approximately 5 million tons, with an estimated sales value of €8.5 billion. The growth rate of the pet food industry has been 3% between the years 2001 – 2003, which is reasonably good expansion compared to the stagnation or negative growth rates observed in allied industries, such as feed for agricultural species. Pet food manufacturing directly employs 21,000 workers, with a further 30,000 employed indirectly.

The significance of the pet food industry for the total agricultural sector is becoming increasingly important, as the yearly purchase of agricultural by-products in European Union has reached 2.75 million tons (FEDIAF, 2004). Manufacturers must continue to be innovative, as this provides market differentiation and increases sales opportunities.

According to Euromonitor International's research (2006), multiple grocers dominate retail distribution with 45% of the sales, a share that has been stable from 1998 until 2005. Vets and pet shops now account for about a quarter of all sales, with a growing segment seen in distribution through specialist pet superstores, which attained a market share of 10% in 2005 (Euromonitor/ PETS International Magazine, 2006). Retail growth is based on demand for a wider range of pet foods, treats and accessories that only these superstores can offer. Whilst supermarkets don't offer unique buying experiences such as shopping accompanied by your companion animals, some pet superstores do, and additionally offer a range of services to meet your animal's individual needs. The fact that a visit to the vet is typically linked to some medical requirement, mean that the sales of pet products via the surgeries represents the smallest retail channel (Euromonitor / PETS International Magazine, 2006).

While pet food volumes have reached a plateau in Western Europe, the situation in individual member states differs. Customer demands are increasingly orientated toward premium products, treats, and, in the segment of complete diets, towards dry food in dogs. (Figure 1). Similar trends are evident with cat owners.

Figure 1.
Market trends of moist, semi-moist, dry pet food, mixers and treats for dogs in the United Kingdom (PFMA, 2005)

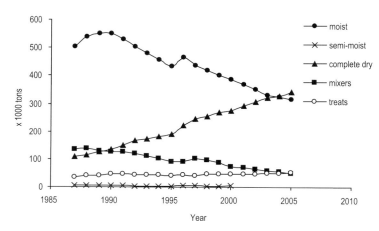

Economic stability in Eastern Europe has been a driving factor for strong market growth in pet food and increased ownership. Lifestyles in certain Eastern European countries have become similar to those in Western Europe, and subsequently purchasing power has increased. Value and volume growth of pet food is in line with the demand for convenience, and an increased understanding of the quality and benefits of prepared food that meets nutritional requirements. Hungary and Czech Republic, in particular, accounted for around one third of the retail sales in Eastern Europe (Euromonitor / PETS International Magazine, 2006).

Consumer expectations

Consumers can be segmented according to income, population growth, urbanisation, age, and household size (PROMAR, 2004). Pet owners have differing, yet specific, expectations that pet food should fulfil, demanding high quality standards in every price segment. Safety, nutritional adequacy and health promotion are important issues. 'Healthiness' is now a major concern for many consumers, especially those who are prepared to pay higher prices for premium products. Other consumer groups expect their pets to derive enjoyment from eating a specific product, or for themselves to enjoy the interaction derived from feeding their pet. Another category of pet owners has been identified as being mainly interested in getting access to lower priced products whilst still expecting nutritional adequacy, as well as high palatability and digestibility of the food.

In many Western European countries, issues have been raised concerning ethical aspects of pet food. Since the BSE crisis, certain raw materials are no longer used by the pet food industry and, indeed, were discarded from the pet food chain earlier than from the human food chain. Ingredients of animal origin must be approved by the veterinary service and be certified as fit for human consumption, otherwise they cannot be used for pet food production. In the higher priced sectors, consumers expect manufacturers to run additional quality controls in their factories to assure optimum quality of ingredients.

Future directions

Future developments are difficult to predict, however it can be assumed that the trends of the last five years will continue, as a considerable number of consumers continue to demand premium quality, and will be prepared to pay appropriate prices. Functionality of certain ingredients in pet food is being investigated, and will result in new products. In this aspect, the European perspective differs from other parts of the world, as the use of dietary supplements in humans is still relatively uncommon. Many comparisons have been made between market developments in human food and pet food. It would be expected that fewer consumers in Europe today are willing to buy functional supplements for their pets. Be that as it may, many benefits derived from functional ingredients can be realised in companion animals. Market potential has already been identified for palatable treats with specific functionality, products with proven efficacy in the promotion of well-being, health and longevity, and foods of 'natural' origin.

Data from Infores (PETS International, 2006) demonstrates the continuous growth of the snack market, with the market value for dog snacks being around six times higher than for cat snacks. Human snacking behaviour in general seems to have been transferred to pets, and snacks and treats are used to facilitate interaction with the animal or as a reward. An emerging market segment in Western Europe is linked to seasonal and holiday occasions, such as Christmas, in the promotion of treats and presents for pets, and is a direct consequence of the continuing humanisation of household animals.

Conclusions

Consumer trends in pet food have evolved dramatically in the last decade, on a global basis. Analysis of specific European changes has shown shifts in the numbers and species of animals kept as human companions, with an increased emphasis on their role as family members. Changes in human society, such as longer working hours, smaller households and increased mobility, can account for these changes and should be monitored closely by manufacturers to allow them to exploit new opportunities within emerging market sectors.

References

Euromonitor (2001). http://www.euromonitor.com/petfood. Accessed 02/22/2004

FEDIAF (2006) http://www.fediaf.org/pages/figure.html. Accessed 08/09/2006

PFMA (2006). http://www.pfma.com. Accessed 08/09/2006

VDH (2006). http://www.vdh.de/cgi-bin/vdh_gesamt/welpenzahlen.pl?sort=2005

ZZF (2001). http://www.zzf.de/presse/markt/markt2001.html. Accessed 02/22/2004

ZZF (2003). http://www.zzf.de/zza/031226.html. Accessed 02/22/2006

ZZF (2005). http://www.zzf.de/dateiarchiv/Heimtierhaltung_in_Europa_2005.pdf

PETS (2005). AC Nielsen / PETS International Magazine, Dec. 2005

PETS (2006). Royal Canin / PETS International Magazine, May 2006

PETS (2006). Infores / PETS International Magazine, March 2006

PET (2006). Royal Canin / PET in Europe 7-8/2006

Promar International (2004). Market Report.

Human consumer trends and elements in pet food

Doerte-Katja Laue

The comparison between pet food and human food

It has been stated that if you see a trend in human food, you will see it shortly after in pet food (PETS, 2006). Market observations and analysis have revealed to the pet food industry that human food and consumer trends give insight into the future demands of pet owners. General buying behaviour is an indicator for what is currently important to consumers, and reflects their interests and beliefs (worldwidebrands, 2006). Pet food producers need to identify such trends and identify how they fit into major social, historical and economic changes (mega-trends) (Horx, 2005).

Pet owners tend to humanise their pets and apply human needs and emotions to their animal companions who live with them at home. Pets can take the position of a full family member and may be treated in the same way as a child, partner or friend. Feeding time is an opportunity for interaction with the pet and marketing e.g. claims on packaging give the meaning to it (PETS, 2006). The pet food industry knows very well that the marketing is aimed solely at the owner, the functionality and nutritional quality being reserved for the animal. Initial communication with the pet owner occurs via packaging and advertising, and has to attract them using familiar phrases, thoughts and beliefs.

Pet owners understand their responsibility for nourishing a pet with balanced food, but they also want to enjoy the feeding occasion. The diverse range of pet food products found in the market today, appeals to many different characters of pet owners, allowing them to select a food they find appealing and deem appropriate for their individual animal. Marketing pet foods to humans, understanding consumer segmentation and tracking trends are the essence of successful sales for pet food manufacturers.

Regional differences

Consumer behaviour and trends are embedded not only in physical, social and temporal experiences but also within historical, cultural, legal and economic contexts. This can be observed in the wide range of consumer behaviours within just one continent, e.g. Europe. Translated into pet food terms; Southern Europe pet food is more colourful and contains (especially in the mid price and economy brands) vegetable kibbles, whereas in Northern Europe pet food is paler and seldom has any vegetable kibbles present. Meat and fish flavour preferences, and their relative sales values, also differ between Southern and Northern Europe.

The global landscape, when mapped by food preferences, shows a wide variety of eating habits in humans (Antonides, 1999). These preferences fall into four main categories: nature, control, culture and enjoyment. Individual countries can be assigned accordingly (figure 1).

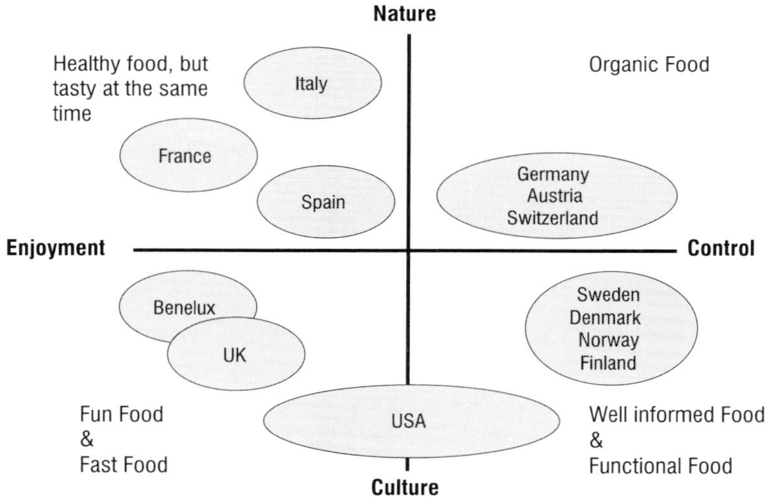

Figure 1. Country landscape as defined by food preferences (GIM argo, 2003)

Healthy food, which is tasty at the same time, dominates markets such as France, Italy, and Spain, where typical Mediterranean preferences for fruit and vegetable consumption are found. Organic food has a higher importance in Germany, Austria, and Switzerland. Source and production processes are often declared on food packaging, with a focus on origination from local farms and traditional food. 'Well informed' and functional foods are more popular in Northern European countries like Sweden, Denmark, Norway and Finland. Food is purchased based on its natural, healthy status, with ingredients legally declared. Fun & fast foods are typically more popular in countries with culturally diverse populations, which may be due to emigration, like the USA, or where cooking habits have been influenced by a history of colonisation, e.g. Netherlands and Indonesia, UK and India (GIM, 2003).

Mega-trends

'Mega-trends' refer to major changes in buying behaviour that change the consumer landscape, and are based both on physiological necessity and external influences (GIM argo, 2006). Mega-trends can influence lifestyles for a long period of time, and may be fundamental in character (Horx, 2005).

Current mega-trends can be identified as:

- **Globalisation**: Many products are shipped within and between countries, with raw materials produced in one country being processed in another. Whilst this seems to offer great opportunities for some people, is may be frightening for others, resulting in an opposite trend arising, e.g. regionalisation (GIM argo, 2006).

- **Aging society**: Social demographics show that larger proportions of the population are now considered 'old', and as a result, age related diseases and longevity have attained higher priority, especially when making buying decisions. Many products are now marketed with claims to preserve youth and fight against symptoms of aging. Increasing elderly populations lead to changes in the composition of households, with an increase in single-person households where pets may feature as a replacement for a partner or children.

- **Smaller households**: The number of smaller households is increasing, due to later first marriages, divorce and more independent elderly people living alone. Coupled with the losses in traditional social communities, more people eat alone and may have a pet for company. The change to fewer people per household appears to be supporting the food trend of personalised nutrition and individualisation (e.g. ready-prepared meals for one).

- **Time constraints**: Time stresses due to longer working hours, shorter holidays and increased mobility has influenced human buying habits. Employment has become less localised, increasing the time required for commuting to work, as well as the loss of local amenities in many regions, which necessitates travel to large centres for shopping.

- **Feminisation**: Women now have more educational opportunities than ever before, which has changed their role in society and made them more aware of nutritional issues. These differences have created opportunities within the workplace, but have also increased time pressure, especially in working women with families to look after. The demand for convenience has been driven by these changes, as purchasing food is still left in the hands of women. Feminisation means also feelings, emotions, intuitions.

- **Time/wealth polarisation**: In Westernised and emerging countries, a major social divide exists between classes in terms of time and money. Wealthy sectors of society tend to have little free time, whereas poorer sectors are time-rich. These changes have given rise to the 'super premium' supermarket brands now available in the market place (Horx, 2005).

Food trends are based on mega-trends, which can drive marketing in different directions. These can include 'retro trends' for e.g. from global to locally-produced foods and from mass market to niche market (Horx, 2005). For a pet food manufacturer, it is very important to monitor mega-trends, as they influence consumer behaviour and living conditions and food trends (Ruetzler, 2005), opening up new areas for marketing and product development not previously available.

Food trends

Close examination of the historic development of food-trends can be used to construct a timeline tracking changes in consumer behaviour (Figure 2). Most of these food-trends were created as a result of a mega-trend, and reflect sociological and historic influences.

Much has been written about food trends. Different nomenclature has been applied to describe different trends, which often vary in number and degree of overlap. Ruetzler (2005) has identified 13 distinct trends found in the food market:

- Sensual food: the enjoyment of taste, smell and visual appearance of the food – slow taste release in the mouth. It covers the new technology of flavour systems and Umami (savoury or flavour-enhanced) taste, but also the conscious eating with taste release in the mouth.

- Convenience cooking: demanded by time issues of time constraints and increased mobility, which has resulted in ready meals becoming important products in supermarket sales. Frozen and canned food features in this group, as does washed and prepared green salad. Personal modification of the ready meal

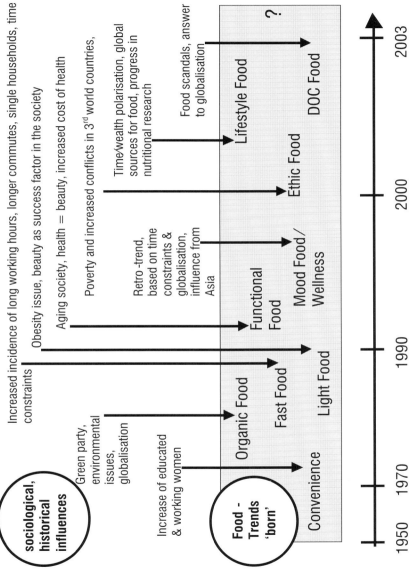

Figure 2. History of food trends since 1950 (adapted from Foodprocessing, 2006) with links to Mega-trends and historical changes and influences

may be included, via some interaction or minimal preparation requirement.

- Fast Casual: combines healthy food from all parts of the world. It fights against fast food and junk food and can be described as the 'fast culinary alternative' e.g. stir-frying, with vegetables and salad as important components.

- Handheld Food: developed for people with limited time, this food can be eaten without cutlery, is the size of an appetizer and fits into one hand. This is the next phase of convenience food, designed specifically to be bought and eaten on the go. It is especially popular with people in the business world, who interrupt the work just for a short while or eat while working at their desk or whilst travelling.

- Health Food: new opportunities for the health-conscious eater. This food category includes salt-, caffeine-, sugar-, fat- and carbohydrate-reduced food, and as it covers the desire to take care for ourselves, it includes aspects of 'wellness'. Nutritional marketing plays a key role within this trend.

- Cheap Basics: these foods focus on price and saving money, and are mainly based on time/wealth polarisation issues. It may be independent of income level, as it also appeals to 'bargain hunters' who derive pleasure from getting a good deal.

- Ethical Food: politically and environmentally sensitive food products. 'Fair trade' or avoidance of child labour may be used in marketing this group.

- Slow Food: a range of food types, which share the characteristics of preserving some type of originality, and reflect the culinary diversity of each region in the world and the preservation of original tastes.

- DOC: 'denominazione di origine controllata' i.e. food is certified as being from a certain original and/or production system. It is the opposite of estrangement and UFOs (Unidentified Food Objects) and fits inline with the registration of product names of specific geographical regions (e.g. Parma ham).

- Natural Food: based on hedonism, moral and politically correct food production. Organic food and livestock husbandry appropriate to the species are key elements within this classification.

- Clean Food: allergen-free, gluten-free, no soya and GMO-free are all claims found on packaging of this type of food.

- Mood Food: the consumption of food as management of emotions or to improve mental performance. The food industry has investigated the impact of food on emotions when it is consumed, for example the change of dopamine and serotonin levels, or effect on concentration and intelligence in school-age children.

● Functional Food: food as therapy, which delivers an additional health benefit above that of the basic nutritional constituents. Claims focus on well-being, overall health and the prevention of diseases.

Further trends linked to human consumer preferences such as 'a kick for the palate' are also known to exist. This refers to the use of specific individual or combinations of spices that give a never-before taste experience, or may feature food prepared in a totally new technological manner. 'Taste fusion' products combine different culinary ideas from regionally diverse recipes to create new 'mouth feel' (Gourmondo, 2006). 'Lifestyle food' reflects the household conditions and personality (GIM argo, 2006). This can be recorded in the increasing sales of 'finest' or 'luxury' brands, as well as ethnic preferences.

Most of these trends can be found in pet food. Table 1 gives an overview of pet products, which are commercially marketed in first world countries. Key trends in petfood are Convenience, Health and Enjoyment / Indulgence, and can be seen as 'cost of entry'.

Table 1. Comparison between human food trends and equivalent pet food products found in marketplaces in first-world countries (Internet research).

Trend	Example of pet food
Sensual food	● Multi textural products, such as crunchy centre with a creamy filling ● Umami/ savoury or flavour enhancing
Convenience cooking	● Frozen dog food ● In general all prepared pet food, some opportunities for personal interaction: ❖ crunch treats to sprinkle dry food on top of wet food ❖ sauces to be added to dry food ❖ dry kibbles with instant gravy poured over
Fast casual	● Introduction of pasta and vegetables to pet food ● Snacks & treats
Handheld food	● Snacks in general ● Copy of human handheld food in treats or food: ❖ Doughnuts ❖ Pizza ❖ Dried small fishes ❖ Sausages in a bread wrapper
Health food	● Light food, ideal weight, calorie controlled ● Vegetarian food ● Food delivered with a measuring cup

15

Table 1.
Contd.

Trend	Example of pet food
Cheap basics	• Private label • Table scrap
Ethic food	• Claim: 'Not tested in animal trials' • Claim: 'Using the most ethical manufacturing processes'
Slow food	• New Zealand: carton of whole meat chunks for cats • Toscana & Ireland variety • Nostalgic food 'for 7 generations'
Certified origin	• 'Taste of Sweden', original from Sweden • With Stockfish from Alaska • New Zealand farm raised meats • Yucca extract from Mexico
Natural food	• Organically sourced raw materials • Free of preservatives, colorants, 'chemical free zone'
Clean food	• Beef free (BSE concerns) • From own trusted suppliers, ISO certified • No soy, GMO-free • Free of allergens • From veterinary controlled slaughterhouses intended for human consumption • Use of beta-glucan
Mood food	• Ingredients like Aloe Vera, Ginkgo, herbs
Functional food	• Beautifying claims • Joint health • Probiotics, Prebiotics • Oral Care • Skin & Coat, organic trace minerals • Immune system, Antioxidants
Lifestyle Food	• Luxury ingredients • Breed specific • Indoor / outdoor • Moulting cats • Coat condition

Most of these trends are combined together when applied to product marketing. Seldom does one pet food product reflect just one trend. It is interesting to note that most of the human food trends have an equivalent in pet food. The strongest trends currently followed include functional food, convenience food, natural food and sophisticated food (which covers trends like certified origin, slow, handheld and lifestyle foods). It can be expected that these trends will become stronger in the future (Goenee, 2006).

Most opportunities available today to pet food manufacturers are based on these trends. The buying decisions made by pet owners are typically based on emotion (Antonides, 1999) and it is of key importance for a pet food manufacturer to be in tune with a customer's decision processes, to motivate them to ensure that they buy the product – in other words to make sure that pet food products reflect the selection processes applied to human food by the consumer.

References

Antonides, (1999) in: *Consumer behaviour: an European perspective.* Eds G. Antonides, W.F. van Raaij New York

Foodprocessing http:// www.itgsalzburg.at/projekte/lmw/ Reichl_Trends_Praesentation_ 06-03-21%20L_ TEC%20 Trends.pdf. Accessed 08/08/2006

Goenee, E.C. (2006) Ed Corrine Goenee, *PETS International Magazine*, March 2006

GIM argo, (2003): http://www.gim-argo.de/ftp/Food_Trends_ Exzerpt.pdf. Accessed 02/02/2004

GIM argo, (2004): http://www.gim-argo.de/ftp/Food_Trends_ Exzerpt.pdf. Accessed 08/08/2006

GIM argo, (2006): http://www.matchmaking.at/food/docs/ gim_de.ppt. Accessed 08/08/2006

Gourmondo, (2006) http:// www.presseportal.de/story.htx?nr = 851734&search =food, trend. Accessed 08/08/2006

Horx, (2005) in *Wie wir leben warden – die Zukunft beginnt jetzt.* Ed. M. Horx, Campus Verlag

Ruetzler, (2005). in: *Was essen wir morgen.* Ed. H. Ruetzler, Springer, Wien and NewYork

Worldwidebrands, (2006): http://www.worldwidebrands.com/pradio/ rssdetail. asp?id =1284

Potential role of yeast and yeast by-products in pet foods

Kelly S. Swanson and George C. Fahey, Jr.

Yeasts in various forms, either whole or as isolates, are used in pet foods for a variety of reasons, including palatability, nutrient sources, to improve the texture or digestibility of the diet or to improve animal health or well-being. Commercial yeast products are now available specifically formulated for use in animal feed and pet food.

Types of yeast

Several strains of the yeast *Saccharomyces cerevisiae* are used in the baking, brewing, distilling, and wine production industries (Sumner and Avery, 2002). Although these strains share common features such as efficient sugar utilization, high ethanol tolerance and production, high yield and fermentation rate, and genetic stability, they also possess properties specific to each group (Trivedi et al., 1986; Benítez et al., 1996). Eight official (plus one tentative) yeast products are currently defined by the Association of American Feed Control Officials (2006), and are differentiated by source of yeast and characteristics such as moisture and crude protein concentrations, and fermentative activity.

Brewers yeast

'Brewers dried yeast' is the dried, non-fermentative, non-extracted yeast of the botanical classification *Saccharomyces*, and a by-product from the brewing of beer and ale. It must contain not less than 35% crude protein and be labeled according to its crude protein content (AAFCO, 2006). As defined, brewers dried yeast must originate from a brewery and the brewing of beverages, beer or ale, for human consumption, and should not be confused with corn wet milling yeast that is used in industrial ethanol production.

Brewers dried yeast and corn wet milling yeast are different in terms of chemical composition and organoleptic properties, which is likely due to differences in the fermentation processes and in the substrates used (Table 1).

In the brewing industry, wort, derived mostly from malted barley, is fermented slowly at temperatures of 10° to 20° C using a batch fermentation process that yields a beer with an alcohol content of approximately 6%. In contrast, during wet milling ethanol fermentation, distillers commonly grind and cook corn by using enzymes to convert starch to sugar. A rapid continuous fermentation process at temperatures between 35° and 38° C then is employed to maximize substrate utilization and ethanol production yielding 9-12% alcohol. Although not fully researched, many of the differences in brewers dried yeast and yeast from corn wet milling ethanol production (e.g., fat content, hops products (caryophyllene, humulene), and sugar profiles) are likely factors that affect palatability.

Commercially available brewers yeast is typically dried from yeast slurry to a dry powder of less than 10% moisture, to facilitate handling, storage, and transport. The product is relatively high in crude protein and carbohydrate concentrations, while the concentrations of fat and ash are relatively low. This is not surprising because yeast synthesizes protein and vitamins while absorbing minerals from the beer wort during the fermentation process. The relatively low fat content of brewers yeast, compared to yeast from commercial wet milling ethanol fermentation, is probably due to substrate differences (e.g. relatively low fat levels in barley compared to corn) and differences in the fermentation processes.

Table 1. Chemical composition of brewers yeast and corn wet milling yeast

Item	Brewers yeast	Corn wet milling yeast
Dry matter (%)	95.3	91.2
Organic matter (% of DM)	94.2	92.8
Crude protein (% of DM)	43.1	46.8
Total dietary fiber (% of DM)	22.5	19.1
Ash (% of DM)	5.9	7.2
Fat (% of DM)	3.0	9.4
Total monosaccharides, mg/g (DMB)	460.8	277.8
Glucose, mg/g (DMB)	369.7	168.1
Mannose, mg/g (DMB)	81.4	60.6
Sugar alcohols, mg/g (DMB)	9.7	49.1
Uronic acids, mg/g (DMB)	7.0	7.2
Caryophyllene, µg/g	0.31	ND
Humulene, µg/g	0.65	ND

Fiber concentration of yeast depends greatly on the method used (Table 2). Although the method of measuring crude fiber (AOAC,

1980) is used for regulatory purposes, results are misleading, as several fibrous compounds are solubilised with this procedure, resulting in a large underestimation of fiber content. The neutral detergent fiber (NDF) method of Robertson and Van Soest (1977) results in solubilisation of viscous fiber components and recovery of cell wall constituents. Because brewers yeast contains a considerable amount of protein that becomes viscous when partially hydrolyzed during the NDF procedure, filtration problems and inflated recoveries result in overestimated fiber concentrations (Merchen et al., 1990). For proteinaceous feeds such as brewers yeast, the method of Prosky et al. (1992) used to measure total dietary fiber (TDF) is most accurate.

Table 2.
Fiber composition
of brewers yeast
(Merchen et al.,
1990)

Item	% (DM basis)
Crude fiber	0.5
Total dietary fiber (TDF)	25.1
Neutral detergent fiber (NDF)	48.2
Acid detergent fiber (ADF)	6.8
Acid detergent lignin (ADL)	2.9

Yeast cell wall

The cell wall of *Saccharomyces cerevisiae* constitutes approximately 15-30% of the dry weight of the cell and consists primarily of mannosylated proteins, ß-glucans, and chitin (N-acetylglucosamine), which are covalently linked with one another. The glucan portion consists of ß (1,3)- and ß (1,6)-chains. Beta (1,3)-glucans, which form the internal skeletal framework of the cell, are the major structural components and are largely responsible for its mechanical strength. This form of glucan is highly branched and possesses multiple non-reducing ends that function as attachment sites for other components of the cell wall (Kollár et al., 1997). Beta (1,6)-glucans are found primarily outside the skeletal framework and often are linked to cell wall proteins.

Mannose polysaccharides are linked to proteins to form a mannoprotein layer localized at the external surface of the yeast cell wall. Two classes of covalently linked cell wall proteins have been identified:

- glycosyl phosphatidylinositol proteins that form a complex with ß (1,3)- and ß (1,6)-chains (Kollár et al., 1997).

- cell wall proteins, with internal repeats, linked directly to ß (1,3)-glucans.

Mannoproteins are strictly regulated in response to changes in external conditions (e.g., heat shock, hypo-osmotic shock, carbon source) and internal changes during the cell division cycle (Horie and Isono, 2001).

While glucans and mannoproteins are main components of the cell wall and found in approximately equal amounts, chitin constitutes only ~ 1-3% of the cell wall. Although present in small quantities, it is a major component of the primary septum and is involved in the separation of mother and daughter cells, making it essential for cell division (Shaw et al., 1991).

Other yeast components

The remaining components of yeast, excluding the cell wall, are collectively referred to as yeast cell extract, and include various nucleotides, enzymes, vitamins, and minerals.

The essential trace element, Selenium (Se), has been heavily studied, as it is thought to play a role in cancer prevention. Selenium is an integral part of the enzyme glutathione peroxidase, which important in the prevention of oxidative damage. In the past, sodium selenite (the inorganic form) was commonly used as the Se supplement for livestock feeds. However, recent studies have identified organic sources (e.g. selenomethionine), that are present in plants and selenised yeast, as more highly digestible alternatives (Yoshida et al., 2002; Gunter et al., 2003). Although growth conditions may influence the proportion of selenoproteins present in yeast, approximately 75 to 85% is in the form of selenomethionine (Ip et al., 2000; Zheng et al., 2000; Yoshida et al., 2002). Other Se forms present in selenised yeast include selenite and selenoamino acids (Ip et al., 2000). The presence of these highly digestible forms of Se may be partly responsible for the beneficial effects observed with yeast supplementation in feed.

Use of yeasts in companion animals

Brewers yeast is used in companion animal foods as a high quality protein source, rich in B-vitamins, amino acids, and minerals. Inclusion of brewers yeast, at 1% levels in companion animal diets, has been shown to significantly increase (P < 0.05) palatability in both dogs (Figure 1) and cats (Figure 2) compared to diets containing 1% wet milling yeast. In these experiments, consumption ratios of brewers yeast were 1.9:1 – 2.1:1 compared to wet milling yeast. In each experiment, a panel of 20 dogs or cats was used to test food preference with a standard 4-day palatability test. Each day on test,

K.S. Swanson and G.C. Fahey

both diets were offered simultaneously for a period of 1 h. To account for right-left bias, the placement of diets was alternated each day. After the 1 h feeding period, both diets were removed simultaneously and weighed to calculate intake.

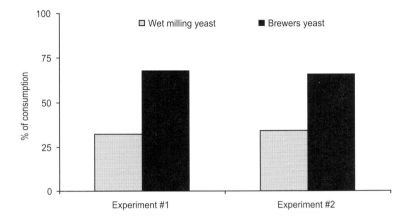

Figure 1. 4 day palatability tests – canine (n = 20 dogs in each experiment). Consumption of dog food including brewers yeast was greater (P < 0.05) than that of a food including wet milling yeast (Kennelwood Inc., unpublished data; Ontario Nutri Lab Inc., unpublished data)

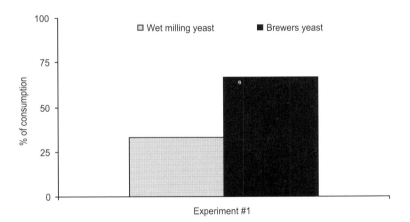

Figure 2. 4-day palatability test – feline (n = 20 cats). Consumption of cat food including brewers yeast was greater (P < 0.05) than that of a food including wet milling yeast (Kennelwood Inc., unpublished data)

Although there are few publications reporting the effects of selenised yeast on companion animal health, one recent experiment studied its beneficial effects on prostate health in aged dogs (Waters et al., 2003). In that study, 49 elderly (8.5 to 10.5 yr), sexually intact males were randomly assigned to one of five treatments and fed for 7 mo; 1. a control diet containing 0.3 ppm Se; 2. control plus 3 μg/kg/d selenomethionine; 3. control plus 6 μg/kg/d selenomethionine; 4. control plus 3 μg/kg/d high-Se yeast; 5. control plus 6 μg/kg/d high-Se yeast. Although no carcinomas were observed during histopathologic examination, Se supplementation significantly decreased (P < 0.001) DNA damage and increased (P = 0.04) number of apoptotic cells in prostate epithelia. Because DNA damage and apoptosis may be Se-responsive events that are important regulatory points in prostate carcinogenesis, selenised yeast supplementation may prove to be protective against its development.

Use of yeast by-products in pet food

'Functional foods', 'nutraceuticals', and 'phytochemicals' are terms commonly used to refer to foods or compounds in foods that possess properties that may benefit the human in ways other than providing nutritive value. Although use of these ingredients began in the human food industry, there is an interest to include them in pet foods as well. Many functional ingredients are thought to decrease the incidence of certain disease states or extend the lifespan of pets by possessing antioxidant activity, antimicrobial action, or immuno-enhancing properties. Several components present in yeast may be classified as being 'functional', including glucomannans, mannans, mannoproteins, ß-glucans, and nucleotides.

Glucomannans

Glucomannans, extracted from the inner cell wall of yeast, may prove to be beneficial in animal foods because of their ability to bind mycotoxins. Mycotoxins are naturally occurring toxic chemicals produced by molds under certain environmental conditions. Sharma and Márquez (2001) tested 12 pet foods commercially available in Mexico for frequency and concentration of aflatoxins. In that experiment, seven aflatoxins and aflatoxicol were detected in most samples, with aflatoxin B_1 being present in the highest frequency and concentration. In all contaminated samples, maize was the main ingredient. Research is needed to measure incidence and concentration of mycotoxins in pet foods commercially available in the U.S., and to determine whether these concentrations are cause for concern. If that is the case, inclusion of glucomannans in pet foods, especially those containing high concentrations of grain, may be prudent. Glucomannans may also play a role in colon cancer prevention because of their antimutagenic and antioxidative activity (Chorvatovièová et al., 1999; Križková et al., 2001).

Mannans

Mannans, also referred to as mannanoligosaccharides (MOS), are composed of short (attached mainly by $\alpha(1,2)$ and $\alpha(1,3)$ bonds and long (attached mainly by $\alpha(1,6)$ linkages by $\alpha(1,2)$ and $\alpha(1,3)$ bonds) chains (Spring and Dawson, 2000). The ability of MOS to agglutinate and interfere with intestinal binding and colonization of harmful microbial species has been studied extensively. Numerous *E. coli* and *Salmonella* strains possess mannose-specific fimbriae, agglutinate mannans *in vitro*, and colonize in lower concentrations in animals supplemented with mannans. Fimbrial adhesins specific for mannan residues are referred to as 'Type-1' adhesins. Mannans aid in the resistance of pathogenic colonization by acting as receptor analogues for Type-1 fimbriae and decrease the number of available binding sites (Oyofo et al., 1989).

Mannans are capable of modulating the immune system and influencing microbial populations in the gut by binding certain bacteria and removing them from the gut microflora. Mannans have been reported to increase ($P = 0.14$) serum IgA concentrations in dogs (2.33 vs. 1.93 g/L, Swanson et al., 2002a). In adult dogs, MOS beneficially altered microbial ecology by increasing ($P = 0.13$) lactobacilli populations to 9.16 from 8.48 $\log_{10}$ colony-forming units/ g fecal dry matter, and decreasing ($P = 0.05$) total aerobe populations to 7.68 compared to 8.67 $\log_{10}$ colony-forming units/g fecal dry matter (Swanson et al., 2002a).

Mannoproteins

Recent experiments have suggested that mannoproteins may be promising vaccine candidates for individuals with compromised T-cell function (e.g., AIDS and lymphoma patients). Mansour et al. (2002) determined that mannoproteins act as ligands for the macrophage mannose receptor, which serves as a link between innate and adaptive immunity (Sallusto et al., 1995). Mannoproteins also have been shown to elicit delayed-type hypersensitivity reactions and induce production of cytokines important in decreasing fungal pathogens (Chaka et al., 1997; Pietrella et al., 2001).

ß-glucans

Although much of the ß-glucan research has focused on oat bran, experiments using ß-glucans derived from yeast have shown similar benefits. Of all the properties reported, the lipid-lowering effect of ß-glucans has proven the most popular. An experiment using obese, hypercholesterolemic men demonstrated that yeast-derived ß-glucans were well tolerated and decreased ($P < 0.05$) blood total cholesterol concentrations similar to the effect of oat products (Nicolosi et al., 1999). Yeast-derived ß-glucans also appear to possess antimicrobial and antitumor properties, due to their ability to enhance immune function. The binding of ß-glucan to the specific receptor present on macrophages results in phagocytosis, respiratory bursts, and secretion of TNF-α (Chen and Hasumi, 1993; Lee et al.,

2001). Finally, ß-glucans are readily fermented in the large bowel and serve as a fuel source for microbial populations.

Nucleotides

Nucleotides are present in yeast extract rather than cell wall. Although endogenously produced by the body, dietary nucleotides may be essential for pets during certain life stages, such as neonates or those with specific health conditions e.g. immune-compromised (Sánchez-Pozo and Gil, 2002). In addition to stimulating the development of the small intestine (Bueno et al., 1994) and liver (Sánchez-Pozo et al., 1998), exogenous nucleotides have been shown to enhance immune function by increasing the production of immunoglobulins, improving response to vaccines, and tolerance to dietary antigens (Maldonado et al., 2001). Because of their importance in neonatal nutrition, the inclusion of nucleotides in human infant formulas is under investigation (Cordle et al., 2002; Ostrom et al., 2002).

In vitro research on yeast by-products

Limited research is available regarding the effects of yeast or its by-products on dog and cat health, with mannans being the only isolate studied to any extent. Vickers et al. (2001) used canine faecal inoculum to determine the fermentability characteristics of MOS. In that experiment, moderate concentrations of total short-chain fatty acids were produced after *in vitro* fermentation for 6 h (0.49 mmol/g of organic matter), 12 h (1.45 mmol), and 24 h (2.40 mmol/g). The microbial species responsible for MOS breakdown were not determined in this experiment.

Hussein and Healy (2001) performed an *in vitro* experiment using canine and feline faecal inoculum to determine fermentability of MOS. Differences were not observed between dog and cat faecal inoculum. By examining dry matter and organic matter disappearance, it appeared that MOS was highly fermented. Dry matter disappearance after 6, 12, 18, and 24 h of *in vitro* fermentation was 54.3, 57.9, 60.7, and 61.3%, respectively. Organic matter disappearance was similar to that of dry matter (56.8, 60.7, 63.7, and 64.1% after 6, 12, 18, and 24 h of fermentation). Dry matter and organic matter disappearance do not always reflect microbial fermentation due to the disappearance of soluble carbohydrates present in the substrates that are not retained during filtering. Although soluble carbohydrates are available for fermentation, gravimetric methods cannot determine the proportion used by the microbes as an energy source. Therefore, the measurement of dry matter and organic matter disappearance is not as accurate as the measurement of the end-products (i.e., short-chain fatty acids and gas), which is directly proportional to fermentation. Concentrations of total short-chain fatty acids, acetate, and propionate increased linearly over time. Moderate concentrations of total short-chain fatty acids (10.1, 26.8, 36.7, and 49.7 mM) were produced after 6, 12, 18, and 24 h. In comparison to total short-chain fatty acids, lactate concentrations were fairly high (7.7, 8.7, 7.6, and 5.9 mM), suggesting fermentation by certain species (e.g., lactobacilli, bifidobacteria). In agreement with the work of Vickers et al. (2001), these data suggest that MOS is moderately fermentable by canine and feline microflora. The fatty acids produced during fermentation suggests that lactate-producing species are able to utilise MOS, which may act as a prebiotic for these species.

In vitro data from our own laboratory indicated that MOS was highly fermentable by canine faecal inoculum (Figure 3).

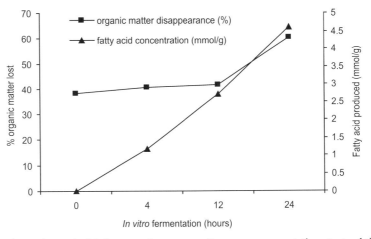

Figure 3. MOS *in vitro* fermentation with canine faecal inoculum (Swanson, unpublished data)

The relatively high organic matter disappearance at the start of the experiment was not due to microbial fermentation, but was caused by the presence of soluble carbohydrates in MOS. Short-chain fatty acid concentrations were approximately twice as high as those reported by Vickers et al. (2001) at the 12 and 24 h time points. In agreement with short-chain fatty acid data, gas was produced in relatively higher amounts (corrected gas values were 17.4, 58.3, and 100.9 mL/g organic matter after 4, 12, and 24 h of fermentation).

Canine research on yeast by-products

O'Carra (1997) performed two experiments examining MOS and its effects on immune function in dogs. In the first experiment, adult beagles were fed diets containing 0, 1, 2, or 4 g MOS/kg diet. Changes in plasma protein and IgG measurements were not observed after 15 or 31 days of MOS supplementation. In the second experiment, Border collie pups were fed diets containing 0 or 2 g MOS/kg. After a 7 day adaptation period, a vaccination protocol was initiated. All dogs were vaccinated against parvovirus, leptospirosis, adenovirus, and distemper. Vaccine boosters were applied on day 21 for leptospirosis, and on day 35 for parvovirus. Blood characteristics were measured over a 9-wk period. No changes were observed in weight gain, lysozyme activity, plasma protein concentration, or plasma IgG concentration. Neutrophil activity numerically increased in pups fed the diet containing MOS following vaccination (approximately 18 vs. 14 Nitroblue tetrazolium (NBT) + cells/slide). However, due to low animal numbers (n = 3), statistical significance was not attained.

Using adult ileal cannulated dogs, Strickling et al. (2000) compared a control diet to those containing 5 g oligosaccharide/kg, one of which was MOS. Researchers measured ileal and total tract nutrient digestibilities, microbial populations, ileal pH, ammonia and short-chain fatty acid concentrations, blood glucose, and faecal consistency. Besides minor changes in short-chain fatty acid concentrations, the only relevant finding was a decrease (P = 0.07) in *Clostridium perfringens* populations in dogs fed MOS (4.48 $\log_{10}$ colony-forming units/g) vs. dogs fed xylooligosaccharides (5.16 $\log_{10}$ colony-forming units/g) or oligofructose (4.74 $\log_{10}$ colony-forming units/g). Because clostridia species do not possess mannose-specific fimbriae, another mechanism is probably occurring. The lack of any significant findings may be due to the low dose of prebiotics consumed (only ~ 1.3 g/d) or the use of soybean meal in the control diet, which supplied an estimated 10 g/kg of naturally occurring oligosaccharides, mainly as galacto-oligosaccharides. Any beneficial effects resulting from MOS consumption may have been masked by the presence of these other oligosaccharides.

Zentek et al. (2002) used 4 dogs in a 4 × 4 Latin square design to determine the effects of MOS, transgalactosylated oligosaccharides, lactose, and lactulose on fecal characteristics, total tract digestibility, and concentrations of microbial end-products in faeces and urine. Carbohydrate supplements were administered daily at a rate of 1 g/kg body weight. MOS supplementation decreased (P < 0.05) fecal pH (6.6 vs. 6.9), faecal ammonia excretion (78.4 vs. 116 μmol/g faeces), apparent dry matter (81.9 vs. 85.0%), crude protein (79.8 vs. 82.5%), and nitrogen-free extract (83.1 vs. 94.8%) digestibilities. By decreasing fecal pH and ammonia, feeding MOS appeared to improve the indices associated with colonic health. However, the decreases observed in apparent nutrient digestibilities resulting from

MOS supplementation would increase faecal quantity and the cost of feeding the animal. The dose of carbohydrate supplements fed in this experiment (1 g/kg BW/d) was very high. Smaller doses of MOS may not have such negative effects on nutrient digestibility.

Using ileal cannulated adult dogs, Swanson et al. (2002a) examined the effects of supplemental MOS and (or) fructooligosaccharides (FOS) on colonic microbial populations, local and systemic immune function, faecal protein catabolite concentrations, and ileal and total tract nutrient digestibilities. A 4×4 Latin square design with 14 day feeding periods was employed, and twice daily, dogs were offered 200 g of dry, extruded, kibble diet and given the following treatments orally via gelatin capsules:

1) control (no supplemental MOS or FOS),

2) 1 g FOS,

3) 1 g MOS,

4) 1 g FOS + 1 g MOS.

MOS supplementation beneficially influenced microbial populations, decreasing (P = 0.05) total aerobe (7.68 vs. 8.67 $\log_{10}$ colony-forming units/g fecal dry matter) and numerically increasing (P = 0.13) *Lactobacillus* spp. populations (9.16 vs. 8.48 $\log_{10}$ colony-forming units/g fecal dry matter). MOS also increased serum IgA concentrations (2.33 vs. 1.93 g/L, P = 0.14) and lymphocyte numbers (20.4 vs. 15.6% of total white blood cells, P < 0.05). A tendency for decreased ileal dry matter (55.0 vs. 67.7 %, P = 0.15) and organic matter (63.6 vs. 74.1%, P = 0.15) digestibility also was observed from MOS supplementation. The combination of FOS and MOS supplementation enhanced immune characteristics, increasing ileal IgA concentrations on a dry matter basis (4.90 vs. 3.40 mg/g ileal dry matter, P = 0.06) and crude protein basis (12.22 vs. 8.22 mg/g ileal crude protein, P = 0.05). Supplementation of FOS + MOS also decreased (P < 0.05) total faecal indole and phenol concentrations (1.54 vs. 3.03 μmol/g fecal dry matter), compounds partially responsible for faecal odor and detrimental to intestinal health. This experiment was performed using healthy adult dogs, which would not be at the highest risk for intestinal irregularities. It is likely that the health benefits of feeding MOS alone, or in combination with FOS, would be most beneficial to elderly dogs, young weanling puppies, or stressed animals.

In a follow-up study, Swanson et al. (2002b) supplemented ileal cannulated dogs with either 1 g sucrose (placebo) or 2 g FOS plus 1 g MOS. Faecal and ileal digesta and blood samples were collected at the end of each 14 day period, to measure microbial populations and immune characteristics. Supplementation of FOS plus MOS increased (P < 0.05) faecal *bifidobacteria* spp. (10.04 vs. 9.42 $\log_{10}$ colony-forming units/g fecal dry matter) and *lactobacilli* spp. concentrations in faeces (9.75 vs. 8.24 $\log_{10}$ colony-forming units/g fecal dry matter) as well as in ileal effluent (8.66 vs. 7.55 $\log_{10}$ colony-forming units/g ileal dry matter). Dogs fed FOS plus MOS also tended to have lower (P = 0.08) blood neutrophils (62.99 vs. 66.13 % of total white blood cells; 6.40 vs. 7.22 x 10^3 cells/µL) and greater (P = 0.06) blood lymphocytes (19.95 vs. 17.29 % of total white blood cells) compared to the placebo group. Serum, fecal, and ileal immunoglobulin concentrations were unchanged by treatment. Supplementation of FOS plus MOS beneficially influenced indices of gut health by improving ileal and faecal microbial ecology and altered immune function by causing a shift in blood immune cells.

Grieshop et al. (2004) tested the effects of chicory and/or MOS on nutritional and immunological characteristics of geriatric dogs. After a 4 week baseline period, 34 senior dogs (beagles: 9-11 yr old; pointers: 8-11 yr old) were randomly allotted to one of four treatments: 1. control (no chicory or MOS); 2. 1% chicory; 3. 1% MOS; or 4. 1% chicory + 1% MOS. Dogs remained on treatment for 4 weeks. Increased (P=0.07) food intake by dogs fed chicory + MOS and MOS alone resulted in higher (P< 0.05) wet fecal output. Dry matter, organic matter, and crude protein digestibilities were unchanged due to treatment. Supplementation of MOS resulted in increased (P< 0.05) fecal bifidobacteria populations and decreased (P< 0.05) fecal *E. coli* populations compared to control. Supplementation of chicory + MOS tended to increase (P< 0.10) neutrophil concentrations, while MOS (P=0.06) and chicory + MOS (P< 0.05) decreased lymphocyte concentrations. Finally, prebiotic supplementation altered proportions of lymphocytes expressing CD4 and CD8 cell surface markers. Chicory + MOS supplementation decreased (P=0.07) CD8-specific lymphocytes. Results of this experiment support findings from previous experiments that in addition to altering gut microbial ecology, MOS supplementation may affect immune status.

Active components in yeast by-products

Our laboratory has analyzed several commercially available sources of MOS and found considerable differences in crude protein, fat, total dietary fiber, and monosaccharide concentrations (Table 3).

Table 3.
Chemical
composition of
several
mannanoligo-
saccharide
sources

Item[1]	Source				
	A	B	C	D	E
DM, %	91.1	92.1	93.4	94.4	96.5
OM, % of DM	91.6	82.2	93.0	93.5	98.1
CP, % of DM	33.7	39.0	34.4	42.2	42.9
TDF, % of DM	37.0	21.4	40.8	NA[4]	NA
Fat, % of DM	6.7	6.1	7.7	6.6	12.1
Glc, mg/g	274.0	214.4	341.6	345.5	188.4
Man, mg/g	119.3	58.6	99.7	90.7	144.0
Gal, mg/g	ND[2]	35.9	ND	ND	ND
Free glc, mg/g	1.8	2.0	1.6	1.8	ND
Free man, mg/g	ND	TR[3]	ND	0.1	ND
Free gal, mg/g	ND	1.1	TR	ND	ND

[1]DM = dry matter; OM = organic matter; CP = crude protein; TDF = total dietary fiber; Glc = glucose; Man = mannose; Gal = galactose.
[2]ND = not detected.
[3]TR = trace.
[4]NA = not analyzed.

Most of the monosaccharides are present as part of polysaccharides rather than as free sugars. Source B was unique in that it contained a considerable amount of galactose in addition to glucose and mannose. The presence of galactose may suggest that guar gum or locust bean gum, which contain galactomannans, are also present in this type of MOS. Although marketed as a source of MOS, these products are very complex and also contain glucans, mannoproteins, phosphate, and several other compounds, which apparently are not excluded in the crude extraction process. Because the composition of MOS is complex, the components that result in beneficial effects are not known. Although the mannan portion of MOS is generally thought to be responsible for the pathogenic resistance effect by acting as a receptor analog for Type-1 fimbrial adhesions present on species such as *E. coli* and *Salmonella*, it is possible that a different fraction present in MOS is responsible for its effects on immune function. For example, mannoproteins and ß-glucans taken from yeast cell walls have been reported to enhance immunity. Therefore, more research is needed in order to determine whether bioactive peptides, ß-glucans, mannans, or unknown factors present in MOS are responsible for the immune responses observed as a result of their supplementation.

Conclusions

Very few experiments have evaluated the effects of yeast or it's by-products on canine health, and no experiments have been performed in felines. The limited data collected thus far suggests that inclusion of yeast products in pet foods may support intestinal health. Although brewers yeast often is included for palatability enhancement, its 'functional' properties may be an even more important reason for its inclusion in pet foods. From the limited number of experiments testing MOS, it appears that it has beneficial effects on indices associated with gut health. MOS supplementation has been shown to improve ileal and faecal microbial ecology and enhance immune status. Because glucomannans are able to bind mycotoxins, their presence in pet foods may also be beneficial. However, yeast-derived ß-glucans, mannoproteins, and nucleotides require further testing to determine their potential role in companion animal nutrition and health.

References

Association of American Feed Control Officials: Official Publication. (2006). *Association of American Feed Control Officials*, West Lafayette, IN.

AOAC. (1980). Official Methods of Analysis. (13th Ed.). *Association of Official Analytical Chemists*, Washington, DC.

Benítez, T., J. M. Gasent-Ramírez, F. Castrejón, and A. C. Codón. (1996). Development of new strains for the food industry. *Biotechnol. Prog.* **12**: 149-163.

Bueno, J., M. Torres, A. Almendros, R. Carmona, M. C. Nunez, A. Rios, and A. Gil. (1994). Effect of dietary nucleotides on small intestinal repair after diarrhoea. Histological and ultra structural changes. *Gut* **35**: 926-933.

Chaka, W., A. F. Verheul, V. V. Vaishnav, R. Cherniak, J. Scharringa, J. Verhoef, H. Snippe, and A. I. Hoepelman. (1997). Induction of TNF-α in human peripheral blood mononuclear cells by the mannoprotein of *Cryptococcus neoformans* involves human mannose binding protein. *J. Immunol.* **159**: 2979-2985.

Chen, J. T., and K. Hasumi. (1993). Activation of peritoneal macrophages in patients with gynecological malignancies by sizofiran and recombinant interferon-gamma. Biotherapy **6**: 189-194.

Chorvatovičová, D., E. Machová, J. Šandula, and G. Kogan. (1999). Protective effect of the yeast glucomannan against cyclophosphamide-induced mutagenicity. *Mutat. Res.* **444**: 117-122.

Cordle, C. T., T. R. Winship, J. P. Schaller, D. J. Thomas, R. H. Buck, K. M. Ostrom, J. R. Jacobs, M. M. Blatter, S. Cho, W. M. Gooch III, and L. K. Pickering. (2002). Immune status of infants fed soy-based formulas with or without added nucleotides for 1 year: Part 2: Immune cell populations. *J. Ped. Gastroenterol. Nutr.* **34**: 145-153.

Grieshop, C. M., E. A. Flickinger, K. J. Bruce, A. R. Patil, G. L. Czarnecki-Maulden, and G. C. Fahey, Jr. (2004). Gastrointestinal and immunological responses of senior dogs to chicory and mannanoligosaccharides. *Arch. Anim. Nutr.* **58**: 483-493.

Gunter, S. A., P. A. Beck, and J. M. Phillips. (2003). Effects of supplementary selenium source on the performance and blood measurements in beef cows and their calves. *J. Anim. Sci.* **81**: 856-864.

Horie, T., and K. Isono. (2001). Cooperative functions of the mannoprotein-encoding genes in the biogenesis and maintenance of the cell wall in *Saccharomyces cerevisiae*. *Yeast* **18**: 1493-1503.

Hussein, H. S., and H. P. Healy. (2001). *In vitro* fermentation characteristics of mannanoligosaccharides by dogs and cats. In: *The Waltham International Symposium Abstracts*, p. 80.

Ip, C., M. Birringer, E. Block, M. Kotrebai, J. F. Tyson, P. C. Uden, and D. J. Lisk. (2000). Chemical speciation influences comparative activity of selenium-enriched garlic and yeast in mammary cancer prevention. *J. Agric. Food Chem.* **48**: 2062-2070.

Kollár, R., B. B. Reinhold, E. Petráková, H. J. C. Yeh, G. Ashwell, J. Drgonová, J. C. Kapteyn, F. M. Klis, and E. Cabib. (1997). Architecture of the yeast cell wall: ß(1→6)-glucan interconnects mannoprotein, ß(1→3)-glucan, and chitin. *J. Biol. Chem.* **272**: 17762-17788.

Križková, L., Z. Duračková, J. Sandula, V. Sasinková, and J. Krajčovič. (2001). Antioxidative and antimutagenic activity of yeast cell wall mannans *in vitro*. *Mutat. Res.* **497**: 213-222.

Lee, J.-N., D.-Y. Lee, I.-H. Ji, G.-E. Kim, H. N. Kim, J. Sohn, S. Kim, and C.-W. Kim. (2001). Purification of soluble ß-glucan with immune-enhancing activity from the cell wall of yeast. *Biosci. Biotechnol. Biochem.* **65**: 837-841.

Maldonado, J., J. Navarro, E. Narbona, and A. Gil. (2001). The influence of dietary nucleotides on humoral and cell immunity in the neonate and lactating infant. *Early Human Dev.* **65**: S69-S74.

Mansour, M. K., L. S. Schlesinger, and S. M. Levitz. (2002). Optimal T cell responses to *Cryptococcus neoformans* mannoprotein are dependent on recognition of conjugated carbohydrates by mannose receptors. *J. Immunol.* **168**: 2872-2879.

Merchen, N. R., G. C. Fahey, Jr., J. E. Corbin, and D. A. Hirakawa. (1990). Researchers seek best way to assess fiber in dog food. *Feedstuffs.* May 14, 1990 issue, pp. 49-51.

Nicolosi, R., S. J. Bell, B. R. Bistrian, I. Greenberg, R. A. Forse, and G. L. Blackburn. (1999). Plasma lipid changes after supplementation with ß-glucan fiber from yeast. *Am. J. Clin.*

Nutr. **70**: 208-212.

O'Carra, R. (1997). An assessment of the potential of mannan oligosaccharides as immunostimulants. *M.S. thesis.* Nat'l Univ. of Ireland, Galway.

Ostrom, K. M., C. T. Cordle, J. P. Schaller, T. R. Winship, D. J. Thomas, J. R. Jacobs, M. M. Blatter, S. Cho, W. M. Gooch III, D. M. Granoff, H. Faden, and L. K. Pickering. (2002). Immune status of infants fed soy-based formulas with or without added nucleotides for 1 year: Part 1: Vaccine responses and morbidity. *J. Ped. Gastroenterol. Nutr.* **34**: 137-144.

Oyofo, B. A., R. E. Droleskey, J. O. Norman, H. H. Mollenhauer, R. L. Ziprin, D. E. Corrier, and J. R. DeLoach. (1989). Inhibition by mannose of *in vitro* colonization of chicken small intestine by *Salmonella typhimurium. Poult. Sci.* **68**: 1351-1356.

Pietrella, D., R. Cherniak, C. Strappini, S. Perito, P. Mosci, F. Bistoni, and A. Vecchiarelli. (2001). Role of mannoprotein in induction and regulation of immunity to *Cryptococcus neoformans. Infect. Immun.* **69**: 2808-2814

Prosky, L., N. G. Asp, T. F. Schweizer, J. W. de Vries, and I. Furda. (1992). Determination of insoluble and soluble fiber in foods and food products: Collaborative study. *J. Assoc. Off. Anal. Chem.* **75**: 360-366.

Robertson, J.B., and P. J. Van Soest. (1977). Dietary fiber estimation in concentrate feedstuffs. *J. Anim. Sci.* **45**(Suppl. 1): 254.

Sallusto, F., M. Cella, C. Danieli, and A. Lanzavecchia. (1995). Dendritic cells use macropinocytosis and the mannose receptor to concentrate macromolecules in the major histocompatability complex class II compartment: Downregulation by cytokines and bacterial products. *J. Exp. Med.* **182**: 389-400.

Sánchez-Pozo, A., and A. Gil. (2002). Nucleotides as semi-essential nutritional components. *Brit. J. Nutr.* **87**: S135-S137.

Sánchez-Pozo, A., R. Rueda, L. Fontana, and A. Gil. (1998). Dietary nucleotides and cell growth. *Trends Comp. Biochem. Physiol.* **5**: 99-111.

Sharma, M., and C. Márquez. (2001). Determination of aflatoxins in domestic pet foods (dog and cat) using immunoaffinity column and HPLC. *Anim. Feed Sci. Technol.* **93**: 109-114.

Shaw, J. A., P. C. Mol, B. Bowers, S. J. Silverman, M. H. Valdivieso, A. Duran, and E. Cabib. (1991). The function of chitin synthases 2 and 3 in the *Saccharomyces cerevisiae* cell cycle. *J. Cell Biol.* **114**: 111-123.

Spring, P., and K. Dawson. (2000). Utilizing biotechnology to improve pet food quality. *Proc. Petfood Forum 2000*, Watt Publishing Co., Mt. Morris, IL, pp. 123-136.

Strickling, J. A., D. L. Harmon, K. A. Dawson, and K. L. Gross. (2000). Evaluation of oligosaccharide addition to dog diets: Influences on nutrient digestion and microbial populations.

Anim. Feed Sci. Technol. **86**: 205-219.

Sumner, E. R., and S. V. Avery. (2002). Phenotypic heterogeneity: Differential stress resistance among individual cells of the yeast *Saccharomyces cerevisiae*. *Microbiol*. **148**: 345-351.

Swanson, K. S., C. M. Grieshop, E. A. Flickinger, L. L. Bauer, H.-P. Healy, K. A. Dawson, N. R. Merchen, and G. C. Fahey, Jr. (2002a). Supplemental fructooligosaccharides and mannanoligosaccharides influence immune function, ileal and total tract nutrient digestibilities, microbial populations and concentrations of protein catabolites in the large bowel of dogs. *J. Nutr*. **132**: 980-989.

Swanson, K. S., C. M. Grieshop, E. A. Flickinger, H.-P. Healy, K. A. Dawson, N. R. Merchen, and G. C. Fahey, Jr. (2002b). Effects of supplemental fructooligosaccharides plus mannanoligosaccharides on immune function and ileal and fecal microbial populations in adult dogs. Arch. *Anim. Nutr*. **56**: 309-318.

Trivedi, N. B., G. K. Jacobson, and W. Tesch. (1986). Baker's yeast. *CRC Crit. Rev. Biotechnol*. **24**: 75-109.

Vickers, R. J., G. D. Sunvold, R. L. Kelley, and G. A. Reinhart. (2001). Comparison of fermentation of selected fructooligosaccharides and other fiber substrates by canine colonic microflora. *Am. J. Vet. Res*. **62**: 609-615.

Waters, D. J., S. Shen, D. M. Cooley, D. G. Bostwick, J. Qian, G. F. Combs, Jr., L. T. Glickman, C. Oteham, D. Schlittler, and J. S. Morris. (2003). *J. Natl Cancer Inst*. **95**: 237-241.

Yoshida, M., S. Sugihara, T. Suenaga, C. Naito, K. Fukunaga, and H. Tsuchita. (2002). Digestibility and chemical species of selenium contained in high-selenium yeast. *J. Nutr. Sci. Vitaminol*. **48**: 401-404.

Zentek, J., B. Marquart, and T. Pietrzak. (2002). Intestinal effects of mannanoligosaccharides, transgalactooligosaccharides, lactose and lactulose in dogs. *J. Nutr*. **132**: 1682S-1684S.

Zheng, J., M. Ohata, N. Furuta, and W. Kosmus. (2000). Speciation of selenium compounds with ion-pair reversed phase liquid chromatography using inductively coupled plasma mass spectrometry as element-specific detection. *J. Chromatogr*. **874**: 55-64.

Glycomics: putting carbohydrates to work for animal and human health

Kyle E. Newman

Introduction

In October of 2001 bioterrorism came to the United States in the form of letters containing anthrax spores. Imagine a time in the very near future when simply eating a carbohydrate fraction from yeast can protect you from such an attack. It is not as far-fetched as you may think. A recent trial in mice found that mice receiving yeast glucans for 1 week prior to anthrax infection had double the survival rate of unsupplemented animals. As a therapeutic agent, mice receiving yeast glucans had a 90% survival rate compared to 30% survival for control animals (Kournikakis et al., 2003).

In February of 2003, the magazine Technology Reviews identified glycomics as one of the "10 Emerging Technologies That Will Change the World." Glycomics is defined as the characterization of the sugars and the structure of these sugars that make up a cell. We are all aware of the quest to define the human genome (genomics: the full DNA complement) that was recently completed. Many are aware of proteomics, which is the study of the full set of proteins encoded by a genome, but very few people are aware of glycomics. Putting these sciences in perspective, genomics was child's play compared to the undertaking of proteomics, which is dwarfed in comparison to glycomics.

New roles for carbohydrates

At one time, it was thought that there were three main roles of carbohydrates in biological systems. The most obvious role of sugar is as an energy source or storage component for energy reserves. The second function is as a structural component such as cellulose or chitin. The third function seemed to be to confound scientists studying proteins and lipids by being associated with these compounds and subsequently needing to be stripped away in order

37

to truly understand the function of the protein. However, it turns out that the glycosylation of these compounds can define their function or serve to stabilize them. A good example of this stabilization is industrial-grade enzymes, where shelf-life and heat stability have been enhanced by glycosylation of the protein.

Unlike amino acids or nucleic acids that have a certain predictability to their structure, there is no simple code for determining the structure of complex sugars. The biological diversity of these compounds can be easily demonstrated by examining the difference between α-and ß-bonded (1-4) glucose units (Figure 1). When these two glucose units are bound in the α configuration, the resulting compound, maltose, is easily degraded by starch-degrading enzymes found in saliva. Conversely, ß-bonded (1-4) glucose represents cellobiose, a compound that is not degraded by any mammalian enzyme system. This exemplifies the difference in biological activity of the same two glucose molecules bound together at the same site with the only difference being the type of bond between them. Compared to DNA or amino acid linkages, which are somewhat linear, imagine the complexity when you consider that a hexose molecule (like glucose) has six binding sites, can branch and the bonds can orient in different ways (as seen in Figure 1). The possibilities for oligo- or polysaccharides can be a bit overwhelming.

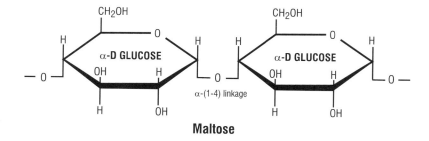

Figure 1.
α- and ß-bonded (1-4) glucose units

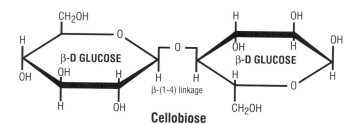

Complex carbohydrates have become a prominent research topic with the realization that distinct carbohydrate structures can have very specific biological activities. One need only imagine the diverse nature of carbohydrate chemistry to understand that the opportunities for novel compounds with unique biological activity are boundless. In fact, the diversity and complexity of these compounds has kept investigators from fully understanding them until recently. Carbohydrates and oligosaccharides are also now being utilized as a nutritional means of enhancing immune function.

Trehalose is a disaccharide of two glucose molecules linked by $\alpha(1,1)$ linkages (Figure 2). This compound is a non-reducing sugar that does not react with amino acids or proteins, making it unaffected by Maillard reactions. When incorporated into materials prior to freezing, trehalose has shown an ability to prevent ice crystallization damage to the molecule. This phenomenon has been exploited to increase the shelf life of materials ranging from foods to probiotic preparations. The role of trehalose is not limited to extending shelf life. It has been shown that mice supplemented with 2% trehalose had reduced symptoms of Huntington disease (Tanaka et al., 2004). Huntington's disease is a rare, hereditary neurological illness characterized by sporadic and involuntary muscle movements. The disease affects approximately 1 in 10,000 people.

Figure 2. Trehalose, a non-reducing disaccharide

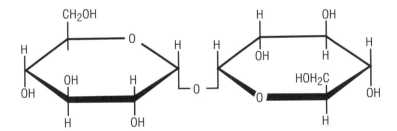

Trehalose has also been examined as a possible therapy in osteoporosis. Ovariectomized mice receiving 100 mg/kg of trehalose had suppressed osteoclast differentiation compared to unsupplemented ovariectomized mice. The improved osteoclast differentiation from bone marrow in supplemented mice prevented the femoral bone loss that is normally attributed to estrogen deficiency (Nishizaki et al., 2000). The most striking finding of this study is that the improvements seen were not due to boosting estrogen levels (the normal therapy for menopause-induced osteoporosis). This could be of enormous benefit since the usual therapy to prevent osteoporosis is supplemental estrogen, which has been linked with certain cancers (Stalhberg et al., 2004).

Carbohydrate-related diseases

The role of carbohydrates in health and disease is coming out of a blur and into focus, but we are only observing the infancy of this field of study. In 2002, a Harvard researcher proposed that an immune response to the complex carbohydrate glycosaminoglycan (GAG) is a potential cause of rheumatoid arthritis (Wang and Roehrl, 2002). Rheumatoid arthritis is a systemic autoimmune disease of connective tissue; and GAGs are a major component of that tissue. This study was unique in that it demonstrated a direct link between human disease, carbohydrate antigens and the immune system.

Congenital disorders of glycosylation (CDG), also known as 'carbohydrate-deficient glycoprotein syndrome,' are a group of inherited disorders where many glycoproteins are deficient in the carbohydrate fraction of the compound. Adults and children with CDG have varying degrees of disabilities such as speech and cognitive difficulties, poor balance and impaired motor skills. Several human diseases are a result of faulty carbohydrate metabolism, the most common of these being diabetes, a condition characterized by abnormally high levels of blood glucose from a failure in glucose transport from the blood into the cells. Another condition related to errors in carbohydrate metabolism is Tay-Sachs disease, an inherited disorder caused by a recessive defect in the gene encoding for hexosaminidase A. This leads to an unusual accumulation of ganglioside GM2 in the central nervous system. Characteristics of the disease include blindness, seizures, a degeneration of motor and mental function with early death in childhood. While most of the defined diseases of sugar metabolism are relatively rare, many of the so-called genetic diseases with unknown causes may be caused by errors in glycosylation because of the importance of glycosylation in cell-to-cell interaction and the role of glycomics in the immune system.

Carbohydrates, cell-to-cell communications and defense against pathogens

Carbohydrates are important surface entities of animal cells that function in a variety of ways to influence cell-to-cell communication, impact the immune system and allow bacterial attachment to the host. These complexed molecules project from the cell surface and form the antigenic determinants of certain cell types. One of the classical examples of this antigenicity is blood type in humans. The ABO blood group antigens are glycoproteins on red blood cells. Small differences in the terminal sugar residues distinguish the A and B blood-group antigens (Kuby, 1994; Figure 3). In addition, mannose binding protein (MBP) is an integral part of the immune system. MBP in the serum can bind to terminal mannose groups on the surface of bacteria and interact with two serine proteases (MASP and MASP2), which ultimately lead to antibody independent activation of the classical pathway of the immune system (Roitt et al., 1998).

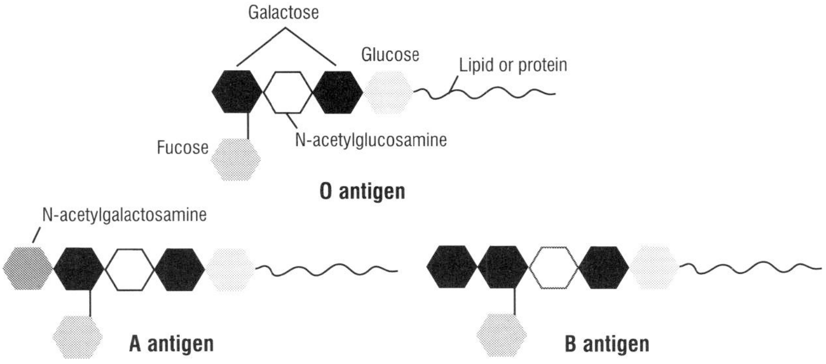

Figure 3.
Differences in the terminal sugar residues distinguish the A and B blood group antigens

Bacterial infection is due in many cases to the ability of the bacteria to recognize host cell surface sugars and use specific receptors that allow them to attach, colonize, and in the case of pathogens, cause disease in the animal. Mannose-specific adhesins (the binding entity on the surface of bacterial cells) are utilized by many gastrointestinal pathogens as a means of attachment to the gut epithelium. One way to prevent pathogens from causing disease is to prevent them from attaching to the epithelial cells in the gut. Early studies using mannose in the drinking water of broiler chicks demonstrated that this therapy could reduce colonization rate of Salmonella typhimurium. Purified mannose and a complex sugar called mannan oligosaccharide (MOS) have been successfully used to prevent bacterial attachment to the host animal by providing the bacteria a mannose-rich receptor that serves to occupy the binding sites on the bacteria and prevent colonization in the animal.

Several studies have been conducted examining the role of mannans and their derivatives on binding of pathogens to epithelial cells in the gastrointestinal tract. E. coli with mannose-specific lectins did not attach to mammalian cells when mannose was present (Salit and Gotschlich, 1977). Spring and coworkers (2000) used a chick model to demonstrate that MOS (Bio-Mos®) could significantly reduce the colonization of Salmonella and E. coli. Animal trials in other species show similar benefits in reducing pathogen concentrations. In dogs, as well as in poultry, reductions in fecal clostridial concentrations have also been noted with Bio-Mos® supplementation (Finucane et al., 1999; Strickling, 1999).

Fructo-oligosaccharides (FOS) have been investigated for nutritional manipulation of the gastrointestinal tract to inhibit pathogens. The principle behind the use of FOS involves the structure and bonding of the fructose molecules. Purified preparations of FOS have been shown to provide a nutrient source for beneficial bacteria such as bifidobacteria and certain lactobacilli. By supporting the growth of the beneficial bacteria it is thought that this will provide an in situ competitive exclusion (CE) effect, thus improving animal health. However, it seems important that the concentration of noncomplexed fructose molecules be kept to a minimum in order for this oligosaccharide to be successful. Oyarzabal and coworkers (1995) found that Salmonella spp. could not use a purified FOS preparation for growth but were able to utilize a commercial preparation of FOS. The authors suggest the use of lactic acid bacteria in combination with FOS as a feasible approach to control Salmonella. Other studies have demonstrated a reduction in Salmonella concentrations in birds challenged with S. typhimurium with and without FOS and a CE culture. FOS alone had little effect on Salmonella exclusion when FOS was administered after infection, but FOS in combination with a defined CE product had an additive effect on Salmonella exclusion especially when used as a prophylactic prior to infection (Bailey et al., 1991). However consistent response of animals to FOS supplementation is a problem and may affect other as yet undefined interactions. Waldroup and coworkers (1993) found that supplementing broilers with 0.375% FOS had few consistent effects on production parameters or carcass Salmonella concentrations. These authors also caution of possible antagonism between FOS and BMD.

Human data for FOS are much more consistent. Hidaka et al. (1986) found that consumption of 8 g FOS/day increased numbers of bifidobacteria, improved blood lipid profiles and suppressed putrefactive substances in the intestine.

Glycomics also plays a vital role in viral diseases. The influenza virus infects by first attaching to a cell surface carbohydrate called sialic acid. This attachment 'opens the door' of the cell and allows the virus to replicate within. The commercial drugs Tamiflu and Relenza shorten the duration of the flu by binding to the active site of an enzyme produced by the virus that frees the virus from the sialic acid. By tying up this enzyme, the virus cannot easily spread and infect other cells (Schmidt, 2002). There are also data examining a novel anti-human immunodeficiency virus (HIV) protein. This protein, called actinohivin, binds to a glycoprotein on various HIV strains and simian immunodeficiency virus (SIV) inhibiting viral entry into cells by binding to this envelope glycoprotein. Further investigation showed that only yeast mannan can inhibit the binding of actinohivin to these viruses. These results demonstrate that the mannose saccharide chains of the virus glycoprotein are the molecular targets of the anti-HIV activity of actinohivin (Chiba et al., 2004).

Sulfated galactomannans also demonstrate in vitro and in vivo activity against the flaviviruses, yellow fever virus and dengue virus (Ono et al., 2003). West Nile virus has also gained a strong foothold in the United States, affecting birds, horses and man. N-linked sugars with mannose residues on the cell membrane protein were found to be important in West Nile virus binding to the cell (Chu and Ng, 2003).

The future of the science of glycomics seems enormous at this time. While mannanoligosaccharide is currently being used to improve health and production of animals, there are enormous possibilities to use other sugars as possible agents against pathogen infection. Table 1 shows a partial summary of scientific studies examining bacterial adhesins.

Table 1.
Carbohydrate
adhesins of
various bacterial
strains[1]

Bacterial strain	Expressing mannose adhesins (% of adhesins those examined)	Other carbohydrate
Campylobacter coli	0	Glucose
Campylobacter jejuni[2]	0	Glucose
Clostridium spp. [2]	0	Galactose, glucose, lactose
Edwardsiella ictaluri	100	Not known
Enterobacter cloacae	100	Not known
Escherichia coli[2]	53	Fructose, galactose, glucose
Fusobacterium spp.	0	Galactose, lactose, raffinose
Haemophilus influenzae	0	Galactose, glucose
Klebsiella pneumoniae	100	Glucose
Salmonella spp. [2]	64	Fructose, galactose
Serratia marcescens	100	Not known
Shigella spp.	75	Fructose
Streptococcus bovis	0	Glucose
Streptococcus suis	0	Galactose

[1] Summarized from Mirelman et al., 1980; 1986; Ofek et al., 2003
[2] In vivo data have shown reductions in these populations with Bio-Mos®.

Conclusions

To say that carbohydrates are involved in virtually every aspect of biology is not an understatement. Finding ways to exploit this knowledge is the current challenge. The vast array of possibilities that exist with polysaccharide structure and function make glycomics a science that may well pass on to future generations. We have only scratched the surface, but we have a better understanding of arthritis, how the immune system works in identifying invasion, how certain congenital disorders debilitate and we have used our limited knowledge to take advantage of the 'sweet tooth' of pathogens to control infection. It brings a whole new meaning to 'a spoonful of sugar helps the medicine go down'.

References

Bailey, J.S., L.C. Blankenship and N.A. Cox. (1991). Effect of fructooligosaccharide on Salmonella colonization of the chicken intestine. *Poultry. Sci.* **70**: 2433-2438.

Chiba, H., J. Inokoshi, H. Nakashima, S. Omura and H. Tanaka. (2004). Actinohivin, a novel anti-human immunodeficiency virus protein from an actinomycetes, inhibits viral entry to cells by binding high-mannose type sugar chains of gp120. Biochem. *Biophys. Res. Comm.* **316**: 203-210.

Chu, J.J. and M.L. Ng. (2003). Characterization of a 105-kDa plasma membrane associated glycoprotein that is involved in West Nile virus binding and infection. *Virology.* **312**: 458-469.

Finucane, M.C., K.A. Dawson, P. Spring, K.E. Newman. (1999). The effect of mannan oligosaccharide on the composition of the microflora in turkey poultries. *Poultry Sci.* **78** (Suppl. 1):77.

Hidaka, H., T. Takizawa, T. Tokunaga, and Y. Tashiro. (1986). Effects of fructooligosaccharides on intestinal flora and human health. *Bifidobacteria Microflora.* **5**: 37-50.

Kournikakis, B., R. Mandeville, P. Brousseau and G. Ostroff. (2003). Anthrax-protective effects of yeast ß(1,3) glucans. *Med. Gen. Med.* **5**: 1-5.

Kuby, J. (1994). In: Immunology. 2nd Edition. W.H. Freeman and Co. New York.

Mirelman, D., G. Altmann, and Y. Eshdat. (1980). *J. Clinical Microbiol.* **11**: 328-331.

Mirelman, D. and I. Ofek. (1986). Introduction to microbial lectins and agglutinins. In: *Microbial Lectins and Agglutins-Properties and Biological Activity.* (D. Mirelman, ed). John Wiley & Sons, Inc. NY.

Nishizaki, Y., C. Yoshizane, Y. Toshimori, N. Arai, S. Akamatsu, T. Hanaya, S. Arai, M. Ikeda and M. Kurimoto. (2000). Disaccharide-trehalose inhibits bone resorption in ovariectomized mice. *Nut. Res.* **20**: 653-664.

Ofek, I., D.L. Hasty, R.J. Doyle. (2003). In: *Bacterial Adhesion to Animal Cells and Tissues.* ASM Press. Washington, D.C.

Ono, L., W. Wollinger, I.M. Rocco, T.L. Coimbra, P.A. Gorin, M.R. Sierakowski. (2003). In vitro and in vivo antiviral properties of sulfated galactomannans against yellow fever virus (BeH111 strain) and dengue 1 virus (Hawaii strain). *Antiviral Res.* **60**: 201-208.

Oyarzabal, O.A., D.E. Conner, and W.T. Blevins. (1995).

Fructooligosaccharide utilization by Salmonellae and potential direct-fed-microbial bacteria for poultry. *J. Food Prot.* **58**: 1192-1196.

Oyofo, B.A., J.R. DeLoach, D.E. Corrier, J.O. Norman, R.L. Ziprin, and H.H. Mollenhauer. (1989)a. Prevention of Salmonella typhimurium colonization of broilers with D-mannose. *Poultry Sci.* **68**: 1357-1360.

Roitt, I., J. Brostoff, and D. Male. (1998). In: *Immunology. 5th Edition*. Mosby International Ltd. London.

Salit, I.E. and E.C. Gotschlich. (1977). J. Exp. Med. **146**: 1182-1194.

Schmidt, K. (2002). Sugar rush. *New Scientist.* **176**: 34-38.

Spring, P., C. Wenk, K.A. Dawson, and K.E. Newman. (2000). The effects of dietary mannan oligosaccharide on cecal parameters and the concentrations of enteric bacteria in the ceca of Salmonella-challenged broiler chicks. *Poult. Sci.* **79**: 205-211.

Stahlberg, C., A.T. Pedersen, E. Lynge, Z.J. Andersen, N. Keiding, Y.A. Hundrup, E.B. Obel, B. Ottesen. (2004). Increased risk of breast cancer following different regimens of hormone replacement therapy frequently used in Europe. *Int. J. Cancer.* **109**: 721-727.

Strickling, J.A. (1999). Evaluation of oligosaccharide addition to dog diets: Influence on nutrient digestion and microbial populations. *Masters Thesis. University of Kentucky.*

Tanaka, M., Y. Machida, S. Niu, T. Ikeda, N.R. Jana, H. Doi, M. Kurosawa, M. Nekooki and N. Nukina. (2004). Trehalose alleviates polyglutamine-mediated pathology in a mouse model of Huntington disease. *Nat. Med.* **10**: 148-154.

Waldroup, A.L., J.T. Skinner, R.E. Hierholzer, P.W. Waldroup. (1993). An evaluation of fructooligosaccharide in diets for broiler chickens and effects on salmonellae contamination of carcasses. *Poult. Sci.* **72**: 643-650.

Wang, J.Y. and M.H. Roehrl. (2002). Glycosaminoglycans are potential cause of rheumatoid arthritis. *Proc. Natl. Acad. Sci. USA.* **99**: 14362-14367.

Prebiotics in companion animals

C. Wenk

Introduction

Companion animal health is linked to many factors, not least being the maintenance of gut function and environment. The last decade has provided useful research into this area, allowing nutritionists to use commercial products to help establish and maintain the gut environment. This is essential if an animal is to maximise the nutrients available from its food and limit the potential for pathogenic bacteria to invade and cause disease. The following review discusses those elements important to gut health, and how certain ingredients such as prebiotics, can be exploited for the companion animal sector.

Eubiosis

A key factor in animal health is the status of eubiosis, i.e. the establishment and maintenance of a stable and healthy microflora in the digestive tract. Eubiosis can be broken down into several areas: digestion of nutrients, vitamin synthesis, stimulation of the immune system (e.g. IgA), protection/strengthening of mucosa as a barrier to invasion and antagonistic effects against pathogenic micro-organisms. In mammals, including companion animal species, eubiosis is initiated by maternal colostrum and milk supply (Figure 1). Early nutritional experiences, exposure to disease organisms and exploration of the environment contribute to the intake and establishment of the gut bacteria. Subsequent nutrition for the rest of its life dictates changes in eubiotic status, including the establishment or prevention of digestive disorders. If feed additives, such as fibre sources (prebiotics), enzymes, probiotics (bacterial cultures), botanicals or acids, are used in feed formulations, they can impact the resident microbial profile, resulting in benefits for the animal.

47

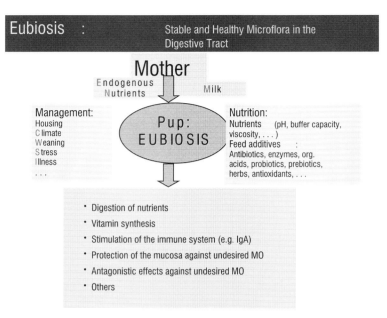

Figure 1.
Factors affecting eubiosis in young mammals

Digestion in pets

The digestive tract in the cat and dog is remarkably similar, given the differences in their eating preferences (Figure 2).

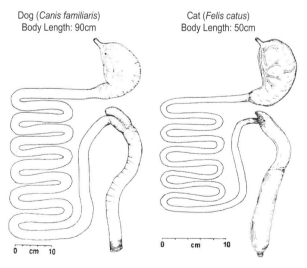

Figure 2.
Digestive tracts of cats and dogs (C.E. Stevens, 1990)

Once consumed, food moves through the stomach, where digestion is initiated, into the small intestine, the major site of digestion via endogenous enzyme secretions, to the large intestine, where bacterial numbers are much higher than in the upper digestive tract and assist in the breakdown of remaining fibre and any other remaining organic matter. The microbial profile of the pig has been extensively researched, and is considered comparable with that of the dog. Dominant species of bacteria on the hind gut tend to be the anaerobes, i.e those that survive in an oxygen-free environment. During early growth and development, the bacteria the animal ingests from its food and environment establish themselves in ecological niches within its digestive tract, where they may contribute positively to digestion and the manufacture of essential nutrients such as vitamins (Figure 3).

Figure 3. Composition and health effects in predominant human faecal bacteria

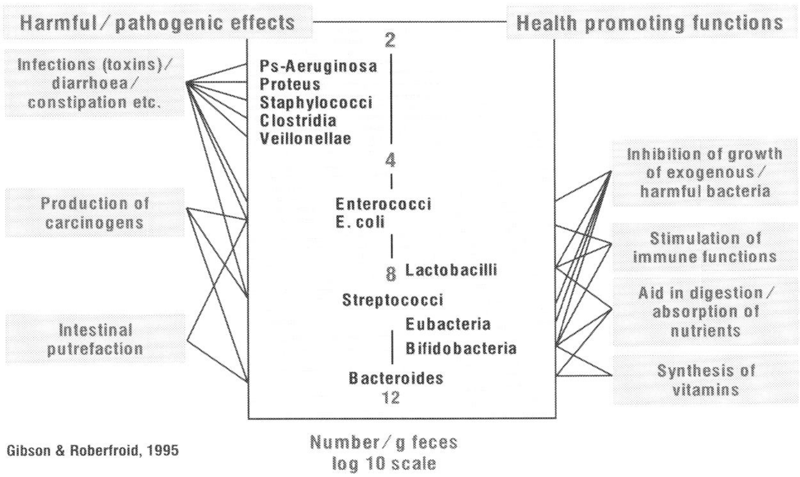

Prebiotics and competitive exclusion

Competitive exclusion is a term used to describe the inability of one bacterial population to establish in the gut due to the presence of another. This principle is used to influence a situation which favours a more desirable microbial profile in the gut. The already-established bacterial populations in the gut have some ability to resist invasion by pathogenic species, by modification of bile salts, induction of immune processes, stimulation of peristalsis, competition for limiting nutrients and substrates (mainly carbon and nitrogen sources and minerals), secretion of anti-microbial substances (ammonia, enzymes, hydrogen peroxide) and competition for receptor sites on the gut wall. The mixture of bacteria and digesta and its activity also creates a restrictive environment for other invading species by altering pH, increasing organic acid concentration and producing compounds such as hydrogen sulphide.

Since the early 1990's certain carbohydrates have been identified which can block bacterial attachment to the gut wall. This is an important factor, as bacteria typically require immobilisation (to prevent them being swept out with the digesta) and to allow them to reproduce. Attachment via lectins is a strategy employed by many pathogenic strains, whereby the micro-organism recognises and binds to the gut surface lectins by way of type-1 fimbrae. It is now well documented that supplementing animals with decoy carbohydrates, such as mannan-oligosaccharides from yeast, results in the binding of such bacteria, and their removal from the gut. This allows proliferation of beneficial bacteria required for efficient digestion.

Pronutrients and eubiosis

Pronutrients are ingredients which promote health and growth in animals above that which is supplied from basic dietary formulations. They include enzymes, organic acids, probiotics, prebiotics, botanical extracts and fibre. Probiotics contain bacteria and which are fed in order to repopulate the gut with beneficial organisms. Prebiotics include non-digested ingredients which can either feed the desirable bacteria (e.g. fructo-oligosaccharides 'FOS') increasing their competitiveness against pathogens, or can bind pathogenic species (e.g. mannan-oligosaccharides 'MOS') removing them from the gut environment.

Fructo-oligosaccharides

FOS is found in artichokes, endives, onions, garlic and asparagus. It can also be produced commercially specifically for in-feed applications. Research has shown that FOS is indigestible by an animal's own natural enzymes, and is selectively used as a substrate by certain bacteria. Detailed trials examining the effects on microflora profile have shown that FOS supplementation increases bifidiobacter and bacterioides numbers and reduces pathogens, with a concurrent drop in ammonia and putrefaction metabolites. Trials with dogs and cats receiving FOS have shown improved levels of beneficial bacteria and reductions in potential pathogens (Table 1 and 2) in faecal samples (Terada *et al.*, 1992; 1993). Furthermore, a noticeable reduction in faecal odour for the animals fed FOS was reported.

Table 1.
Effect of FOS on gut bacteria in dogs (Terada *et al.*, 1992)

Diet	Bifidiobacter (per g dry faeces)	Clostridia perfringens (per g dry faeces)
Control	3.1×10^9	3.9×10^9
FOS (1.5 g/d)	3.9×10^{10}	1.1×10^5

Table 2.
Effect of FOS on
gut bacteria in
cats (Terada *et al.*, 1993)

Diet	Bifidiobacter (per g dry faeces)	Lactobacilli (per g dry faeces)
Control	Not detected	1.3×10^9
FOS (1.5 g/d)	4.6×10^9	4.0×10^{10}

The impact that improving microflora profile can have on digestion and uptake of nutrients (minerals in this case) was demonstrated in another feeding trial (Beynen *et al.*, 2002) where dogs fed FOS had significantly higher levels of mineral absorption (Table 3).

Table 3.
Effect of feeding FOS on mineral absorption in dogs (Beynen *et al.*, 2002)

Mineral (apparent absorption as % of intake)	Control	FOS (10 g/d)
Calcium	8.6b	16.0a
Magnesium	14.0b	23.4a
Phosphorous	26.6	29.5

Means not sharing a letter differ significantly

Mannan-oligosaccharides

MOS, as previously discussed, has a completely different mode of action to FOS. Figure 4 illustrates how MOS binds to pathogens, effectively eliminating them from the gastro-intestinal tract. In addition, immune benefits have been identified in animals fed MOS-supplemented diets. This is thought to be due to the interaction between these types of carbohydrates and the gut-associated lymphatic tissue (GALT), which responds to carbohydrate attachment and the improved presentation of pathogens facilitated by MOS.

Figure 4.
Bacterial binding by carbohydrates and lectins (Sharon & Lis, 1993)

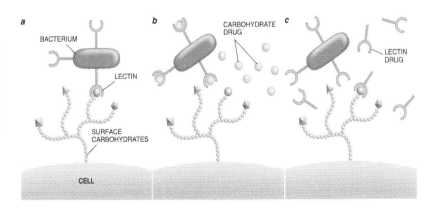

51

The binding efficacy of a commercial yeast-derived MOS product (Bio-Mos®, from Alltech®) on bacterial species such as Salmonella and *E. coli* has been demonstrated in many trials on avian and mammalian species.

Prebiotic synergy

Specific research with dogs has shown that FOS and Bio-Mos®, in combination, result in a synergistic effect, whereby microbial populations and immune responses are enhanced (Figure 5 and 6, Swanson *et al.*, 2001).

Figure 5.
Effect of FOS and MOS fed in combination to dogs on faecal bacteria (Swanson *et al.*, 2001)

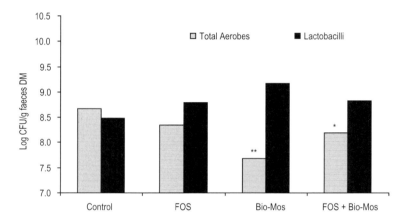

indicates significant difference ($p < 0.05$; **$p < 0.01$)

Dogs fed Bio-Mos® alone had much reduced levels of aerobic bacteria – a classification that includes pathogens. The beneficial lactobacilli, conversely, increased in numbers. Overall both FOS and Bio-Mos® improved the microflora of the gut relative to the control diet.

Figure 6.
Effect of FOS and Bio-Mos® on ileal IgA immunoglobulins in dogs (Swanson *et al.*, 2001)

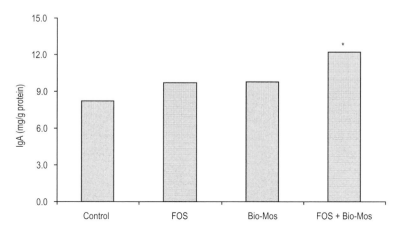

*indicates significant difference ($p < 0.01$)

The importance of using an appropriate carbohydrate has been demonstrated by comparison trials on faecal moisture in dogs (Strickling *et al.*, 2000) where three types of oligosaccharides were studied (Figure 7). Dogs fed xylose oligosaccharides (XOS) did not show the same benefits as those receiving the FOS or Bio-Mos® treatments.

Figure 7. Comparison of three types of oligosaccharides on dog faecal moisture (Strickling *et al.*, 2000).

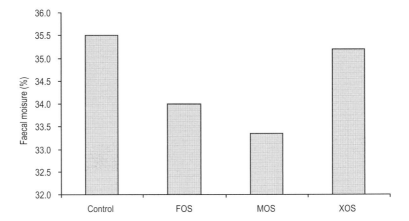

Unlike many agricultural species, faecal smell is important in companion animals, especially cats that use litter trays in the house. Improving the eubiotic status can reduce the production of compounds that contribute to faecal smell. Swanson *et al.* (2001) showed, as part of their trials, that feeding FOS and Bio-Mos®, especially in combination, significantly reduced the production of indole and phenolic compounds in faecal material. Likewise, Strickling *et al.* (2000) showed that ammonia levels were reduced by more than 20% in dogs receiving a Bio-Mos®-supplemented diet.

At a more basic formulation level, improvements in insoluble digestibility have been noted when canine diets have been formulated using higher fibre sources, such as sugar beet pulp and soy fibre (Table 4). This is a strategy now employed commercially by several pet food companies, particularly those marketing products for animals with digestive sensitivities.

Table 4. Effect of fibre source on digestibility in dogs (Kappel *et al.*, 1998)

Fibre source	Digestibility (%)		
	Total fibre	Insoluble fibre	Soluble fibre
Control	32.2	11.2b	73.5
Beet pulp	25.8	15.5ab	61.0
Soy bean	25.8	21.9a	59.9

Means not sharing a letter differ significantly

These benefits have been especially pronounced in the presence of MOS, with 18% increase overall in soluble fibre digestion reported for high fibre diets supplemented with MOS.

Conclusions

Prebiotics such as MOS and FOS are useful in establishing and maintaining eubiosis in companion animals. Commercial MOS products such as Bio-Mos® have been shown to beneficially improve gut bacterial populations by increasing levels of beneficial organisms, such as lactobacilli, and reducing aerobic pathogens. The mode of action of this product is also associated with improved immunity, by increasing ileal IgA concentrations.

FOS works in a different manner, and can be obtained commercially via extraction from certain plants. Although research into FOS has shown benefits in bacterial populations, it is most effective when used in combination with another prebiotic, such as MOS. In combination, these ingredients can help maintain gut bacterial profiles and reduce faecal odour.

References

Beynen, A.C., Baas, J.C., Hoekemeyer, P.E., Kappert, H.J., Bakker, M.H., Koopman, J.D., and Lemmens, A.G. (2002). Faecal bacterial profile, nitrogen excretion and mineral absorption in healthy dogs fed supplemental oligofructose. J. Anim. Physiol. Anim. Nutr. 86, 298-305.

Beynen, A.C., Kappert, H.J., Lemmens, A.G., and Van Dongen, A.M. (2002). Plasma lipid concentrations, macronutrient digestibility and mineral absorption in dogs fed a dry food containing medium-chain triglycerides. J. Anim. Physiol. Anim. Nutr. 86, 306-312.

Gibson and Roberfrois (1995).

Kappel; L., B. Henk; P. Jowett and C. Hedhund. (1998). Effect of Mannanoligosaccharide on Diet Component Digestibility and Fermentation Characteristics in Dogs. School of Veterinary Medicine, Louisiana State University, Baton Rouge, LA.

Sharon and Lis (1993). Scientific American 268(1): 74-81.

Stevens C. E. and Hume I. D. (1995). Comparative physiology of the vertebrate digestive system, Cambridge University, UK

Strickling J, Harmon D, Dawson K and Gross K (2000) Evaluation of oligosaccharide addition to dog diets: influences on nutrient digestion and microbial populations. Anim Feed Sci Tech 86:205–219.

Swanson K. S., Grieshop C. M., Flickinger E. A. Bauer., L. L, Healy

H. P., Dawson K. A., Merchen N. R., and Fahey, G. C. Jr. (2002). Supplemental fructooligosaccharides and mannanoligosaccharides influence immune function, ileal and total tract nutrient digestibilities, microbial populations and concentrations of protein catabolities in the large bowel of dogs. J. Nutr. 132(5):980-989.

Terada A., Hara H., Kataoka M., and Mitsuoka T. (1992) Effect of dietary lactosucrose on faecal flora and faecal metabolites of dogs. Microb Ecol Health Dis 5:43–50

Terada, A., Hara, H., Kato, S., Kimura, T., Fujimori, I., Hara, K., Maruyama, T. and Mitsuoka, T.(1993) Effect of Lactosucrose (4,f-â-D-galactosylsucrose) on fecal flora and fecal putrefactive products of cats.J.Vet.Med.Sci.55, 291-295.

Minerals in pet food: adequate versus optimum

John A Lowe

Introduction

Minerals, based on their metabolic role and evidence from other species, are an essential component of the diet for a dog or cat. With only evidence for the essentiality of 11 minerals in the dog and cat, it is not surprising that there is a paucity of information on the bio-availability of minerals and their requirements in pet species. We do have information on the outcome of mineral excess or deficiency, but in terms of optimum nutritional supply, our understanding remains poor. There are two main classes of minerals;

- macro minerals, usually regarded as those whose amounts are measured in grams per 1000kcal

- micro or trace minerals expressed as milligrams or less per 1000kcal. Typically these minerals are found in the ash fraction of a diet as phosphates, carbonates, oxides, sulphates; however the trace minerals iron, zinc, copper, manganese and selenium are found in other "organically" bound forms, often with amino acids, peptides or proteins.

These organic forms have spawned a new generation of research specifically examining relative bio-availability, and in some cases, determining the amounts required to optimise certain biochemical processes, animal well-being, physical appearance or life stage performance.

Optimum versus adequate

The concept of 'optimum' as opposed to 'adequate' has recently come to the forefront of the debate surrounding the level of nutrients best suited for pets. It is now a primary concern for pet food designers, not just from a nutritional point of view but also from a marketing stance.

The underlying concept of 'optimum nutrition' can be found in both the farm animal industry, where it has been extensively developed and applied for vitamins by DSM Nutritional Products (2000) (formerly Roche Vitamins), and for amino acids, and in human nutrition (Strain, 1999).

The idea behind 'optimum nutrition' is that the design of the diet should promote physiological and mental functions and minimize the development of degenerative disease, resulting in long-term well-being, rather than merely overcoming overt clinical deficiencies. The 'optimum level' would therefore provide a route to support all aspects of biochemical, immunological, haematological and physiological quantifiable functional parameters. Perhaps this could be considered as 'adequacy', which may then also constitute a redefinition of 'requirement'. This concept is a much better reflection of what has started to happen to nutrition over recent years, rather than, as many critics have suggested, the concept being used as an excuse for overt or excessive fortification of the diet. Optimum nutrition is not about excessive supplementation or necessarily large increases in nutrient supply and, most of all, not about any one nutrient in isolation; but is about understanding the consequences of small changes and interactions in nutrients. A study by Kealy *et al* (2002) showed that 'optimum' might actually be less rather than more. Their research reports that a reduction in calorie intake led to a lower body mass, increased life span and delayed the onset of several diseases.

Taking the dictionary definition of the words 'optimum' and 'adequate', it is possible to see why a redefinition of 'requirement' may be applicable:

Optimum: most favourable conditions (for growth, reproduction etc.) best compromise between opposing tendencies, best or most favourable (optimum temperature). From the Latin *Optimus* meaning best.

Adequate: proportionate to the requirements for success of fulfilment, sufficient, satisfactory, barely sufficient. From the Latin *adaequatus*, make equal.

In some ways the two terms may be considered the same, or at least one as quantifying the other; the most favourable conditions to meet the requirements for success; although 'optimum' has a better marketing image.

Classically, adequacy would have referred to minimal nutrient requirement and would not have reflected the fact that there is probably more than one 'adequate' level of a nutrient for an animal species. Historically we have considered the level to be that which overcomes overt signs of deficiency and then usually only for adult animal at maintenance. Clearly there will be differences due to life stage (Shields 1998) and other impinging factors. Until recently, differences in optimum or adequate levels were not considered dependent upon the criteria used for measuring them. It is in this sense that 'optimum' becomes the better descriptor as the level that addresses all the important biochemical, immunological, haematological and physiological quantifiable functional parameters.

It is now recognised that the single amount of daily nutrient intake deemed adequate or optimal for one aspect of metabolism may not be for another. Thus the term 'adequate' is used to mean 'minimal' to avoid deficiency in the classical sense, and 'optimal' means 'enough to maximise the metabolic processes' i.e. those considered most important to the animal.

Problems regarding optimum trace mineral levels

The first problem in optimising minerals is the paucity of nutritional research data for companion animal species. As recently as 2002, major gaps in the knowledge of mineral requirements of cats (Fascetti and Morris, 2002) have been clearly identified. Even now with the publication of the new NRC Nutrient Requirements of Dogs and Cats (2006), we have comparatively little new information.

Secondly, it has become increasingly evident that adverse biochemical changes occur before diagnostic signs of trace element deficiencies are apparent (Chesters and Arthur, 1988), thus we need to consider what the best measurement criteria are for the metabolic processes in which our interest lies. For example, when evaluating copper supplies in the cat, the biochemical markers (plasma Cu, superoxide dismutase and cerulopasmin) appear to be unresponsive to dietary copper intake. Similarly studies examining dietary zinc supply indicate differing 'optimum' dietary amounts depending upon whether measurements of growth, bone development, essential enzymes tissue accumulation or immune status are used as the main criteria. There is also an ever-changing understanding of the role of the mineral in the metabolic process, and this in itself may be further compounded by the fact that there may be a point where some other factor becomes limiting, making it impossible to determine the appropriate level for the nutrient under test.

Thirdly, assuming it is possible to determine the appropriate amount of the mineral to feed for the desired response under experimental conditions, extrapolation to practical applications of this value in a commercial diet is fraught with further complications. Not least of these is the relative bio-availability of the precise form of trace mineral to be used in the diet compared to the one used in the study. A further consideration is whether or not the diet, or processing thereof, influences the bio-availability of the mineral, even if it is in the same form as that used in the experimental procedure.

It is known from early classical studies (Dyer, 1969) that over supply of one mineral can interact (often undesirably) with another. This means a blanket over-supply of any one mineral is undesirable in experimental terms, and is also not necessarily effective in meeting nutrient requirements in practical terms (Figure 1). Too much of many trace minerals can cause pro-oxidation under certain conditions, which is also problematic

The chemical form of the mineral is important. Oxides are not only relatively low in chemical reactivity, but also, in some cases, in bio-availability, whereas the sulphates tend to be highly reactive and yet often more available. This has a bearing on the stability of mineral / vitamin premixes. Sodium selenite and selenomethionine are absorbed and metabolised by different metabolic pathways, making comparisons based on absorption and tissue deposition misleading and not directly comparable to utilisation or bio-availability, or, for that matter, on oxidative load and thus the total anti-oxidant capacity of the animal. The availability of minerals during disease is also worthy of consideration. An animal under stress often tries to alter the metabolic availability of trace minerals to influence the outcome of the disease process.

Figure 1.
Chart of mineral interaction adapted from Dyer (1969)

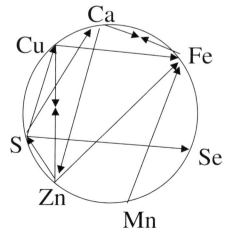

has an adverse affect on

A ————————▶ B

A number of other considerations are important in trace mineral nutrition. It is sometimes inappropriate to extrapolate from one animal species to another. For example, 3, 5 di-iodosalicyclic acid is well absorbed by both rats and cattle, but cattle are incapable of separating the iodine from the organic part of the mineral, so the ultimate utilisation is poor. Two lessons need to be learned from this finding:

1. appreciation of species difference
2. absorption is not always a good indicator of utilisation of a trace-mineral

Other dietary components can influence mineral metabolism. The presence of 2 picolinic acid in the diet increases Zn absorption by 60% in rats but it also increases urinary loss so that the net retention is actually similar.

The future for trace mineral supplementation

Pet foods have been supplemented with trace minerals ever since mineral deficiencies were first understood. The use of conventional inorganic mineral sources has proved both effective and economic, however pet nutritionists have been aware of the problems associated with these mineral sources, which include:

- variability in their bio-availability
- consistency of quality
- possible contamination with heavy metals
- mineral to mineral interactions
- reactivity in supplements and premixes
- the fact that the animal's natural diet trace minerals often exist in complex organic forms

Natural claims are now becoming an important marketing approach in food and pet food, thus to be able to emulate the 'natural' mineral supply with the confidence of bio-availability represents an important step forward in mineral supplementation of today's pet foods.

New information and literature reviews are always welcomed by the industry to help progress such ideas. The new NRC (2006) publication, perhaps the most recent comprehensive review readily available, quite rightly only uses published information in refereed journals. To this end the considerable 'in-house' information of many of the leading pet food companies, research centres and mineral providers are, in many cases, not included in this document.

It is worth noting that between 1974 and 1985 the NRC nutrient requirements of dogs (1985) considered that there was no significant new data that would cause an alteration in the estimated requirement values for minerals. It is also interesting to look at the numbers of animals used to determine the values in early studies. Selenium trials (Van Vleet, 1975) used just 2 puppies in the study, and Se requirements for cats were extrapolated from other species (NRC, 1986), there being no studies on cats at that time. Whilst there are some slight revisions in the new NRC, for example estimates of availability are considered, much of recommended amounts remain based on older data. Some notable changes in requirements and data supply include Mg, Se, Cu and the introduction of safe upper limits. Mineral nutrition is still a relatively unsupported area.

A review of commercial pet foods carried out at the beginning of the 21st century (Table 1) indicated that, whilst there is general agreement on the amount of macro minerals required in the diet, some companies have decided that higher inclusions of the trace minerals offer commercial (nutritional and marketing) benefits. Whether this is due to bio-availability of the supplemental source or for nutritional effect is not immediately apparent.

Table 1.
A comparison of commercial pet foods, standardised for energy and dry matter

Values (%) Macro minerals	Ca	P	Mg	Na	K
Mean	1.4	1.1	0.13	0.37	0.65
Range	0.7-2.4	0.7-1.5	0.10-0.23	0.18-0.60	0.43-0.80
AAFCO	1.0	0.8	0.04	0.3	0.6
Values (mg/kg) Trace elements	Cu	Zn	Mn	Fe	Se
Mean	14.5	222	58	263	0.69
Range	7-26	138-340	15-90	120-476	0.33-1.88
AAFCO	7.3	120	5.0	80	0.11

Bio-availability is often overlooked in formulations. In many cases it is the total content that is met, with little or no consideration for availability of the mineral source or the relative differences in contribution from plant and animal sources. Legislation does not help this situation, as only total content is required for declaration, with no indication as to whether or not this meets requirements (adequate versus optimum). The expression of copper as 'cupric sulphate' is not intended in the legislation to indicate relative availability of the copper present. Copper in plants equates to approximately 50% of the bio-availability of animal sources, and supplemental sources (with the exception of oxides and sulphides which are less available) are similarly absorbed (Ammerman, Baker and Lewis 1995).

It should be remembered that bio-availability is not a single entity but made up of a number of factors which can be expressed by the intuitive equation:

Bio-availability (RB) = fD.E/I.T.Ut

Where fD is the proportion of the dietary supplied nutrient absorbed, E/I the ratio of agonists to antagonists in absorption, transport and utilisation, T is the proportion transported to and or assimilated and Ut is that proportion which is utilised upon arrival at the metabolic site. Note this approach also recognises that the equation values vary for every metabolic site considered.

Specific minerals considered

Copper

Copper supplied in the form of a chelated proteinate, albeit from a limited number of studies in species other than dogs and cats, appears to be better absorbed than copper from an inorganic sulphate source (Ammerman, Baker and Lewis 1995). Differences in availability have been observed for single amino acid chelates, with lysine-copper having relatively higher bio-availability than methionine-copper in chickens. In rats, all amino acid copper chelates have greater relative bio-availability than either animal tissue or sulphate sources.

The work of Dyer (1969) indicates antagonism between Cu and Zn in the diet. Studies in rats (Lowe et al., 1997) indicated that the absorption and retention of copper in tissues is improved when dietary zinc oxide was replaced by a zinc chelate. This may be due to reduced interactions at gut wall or at the mineral transport system level (Table 2).

Table 2. Tissue copper and zinc concentrations in rats on diets containing supplementary zinc from either and oxide or chelate source

| Tissue | Zinc Chelate Diet | | Zinc Oxide Diet | |
	Zinc mg/kg	Copper mg/kg	Zinc mg/kg	Copper mg/kg
Liver	125	33	46	9
Kidney	162	45	27	13
Femur	243	55	120	5

Copper requirements in dogs appear to be low (providing other mineral antagonists are not excessive), at around 3-5 mg/kg diet to prevent anaemia, although there are few deficiency studies supporting this fact. Toxicity has been reported at comparatively low dietary Cu levels, however this is predominately for specific breeds who have an inherited copper storage disease, particularly terriers (Brewer 1998). For the maintenance of coat condition (copper has a key role as an electron donor in the pro-enzyme tyrosinase) higher, and presumably safe levels (as there is no data available on the safe upper limit) are used in pet food, probably resulting from differences in bio-availability of the dietary sources used.

In cats, current NRC (1986) values appear to be marginal for breeding queens, as trials show higher conception rates when fed 10.8 mg/kg of copper compared to those fed 4 and 5.8 mg/kg (Fascetti and Morris 2002). Differences in bio-availability of various forms of copper have been observed in cats (Fascetti and Morris 2002), with copper oxide effectively being unavailable to the cat .

Iodine

Iodine is an essential micro-mineral for all species. It occurs predominately in plant tissue as inorganic iodine and is readily absorbed in the gut. Iodine is not uniformly distributed geographically, with some areas of the world being extremely low, requiring supplementation for diets prepared with local raw materials. However, for cats there is some suggestion that they receive sufficient (even an excess) of iodine in prepared pet food, and would be overdosed if supplemented further (Tarttelin and Ford, 1994). The safe range is reported at [3]6 to < 13.8 mg/kg diet DM basis. The requirement of 220 mg/1000kcal for dogs is usually present in most commercial pet foods.

Manganese

There is very limited work on manganese in any species, and little or no specific studies in companion animals. It appears that methionine and protein-chelated manganese supplements are utilized to a greater degree than sulphates (Ammerman, Baker and Lewis 1995). The presence of cereals in formulations, due to their phytate and fibre content that binds Mn, significantly decreases the already low Mn availability. As little as 1 % of wheat bran and 5 % of a corn / soya mix can cause this effect. A requirement in dogs of 1.2 mg/1000kcal and 1.8 mg/1000kcal for cats is considered adequate

Zinc

Compared to animal tissue (with an index of 1.0), the relative availability of zinc from grains and legumes is typically in the range 0.6-0.7, with some values reported as low as 0.45 for corn. Early studies, comparing sulphates and oxides of zinc, reported similar index values, although more recent studies indicate sulphates to be approaching twice the bio-availability of the oxides. Organic sources have been studied in some detail, and data from poultry suggests comparative values of 1-1.25 for proteinates and chelates compared with sulphates (Ammerman, Baker and Lewis 1995). Wedekind and Lowry (1998) reported that Zn proteinates had a relatively greater bio-availability compared to oxide forms, but commented that, in their opinion, only certain dietary conditions result in organic zinc sources being universally beneficial over conventional sulphate sources. Depending upon the criteria used for measuring the relative bio-availability (e.g. rapidly growing tissue or that with high requirements for the nutrient) significant differences have been observed between chelate, oxide and sulphate sources of zinc (Lowe and Wiseman, 1998), although in this study differences between sulphate and oxide were not found, due to high between-dog variability.

Iron

Practically all of the iron in the body is in the organic form, with only a small amount being found as free inorganic ions. There are two types of organic iron, haem and non-haem. The haem form is present in the porphyrin ring of haemoglobin, myoglobin, cytochromes, cytochrome oxidase, catalase and peroxidase, and represents 70-75% of the total iron content in the body. Non-haem iron is found in transferrin, lactoferrin, ferritin and other iron proteinates. In terms of bio-availability, iron of plant origin is better absorbed than non-haem iron in animal tissue, whereas the haem iron of animal tissue is absorbed as the haem moiety very effectively. The many complex interactions of iron with other minerals, nutrients and food stuffs make deduction of true uptake difficult. Data from studies in rats appears to correlate well with the limited studies in dogs.

In inorganic forms, the ferrous state has a higher bio-availability than the ferric state, benefiting absorption from the acidic reducing environment of the proximal intestine. It is interesting to note that ascorbic acid (vitamin C) reduces and chelates non-haem iron, increasing its absorption. In order for the ferric ion to be soluble, a pH of < 4.0 is required. Since ascorbic acid can improve iron absorption during times of increasing gut pH, it is possible that this may be the principle mode of action of the antioxidant on Fe uptake, and not its direct effect on pH.

The tridentate iron chelates of cysteine, histidine and lysine substantially improve absorption, indicating a relatively higher bio-availability of this mineral from organic sources. Data in pigs (Ammerman, Baker and Lewis 1995) tend to support this, showing that methionine and protein-chelated iron has a greater bio-availability than ferrous sulphate.

Selenium

Selenium is a particularly interesting element, even though limited work has been carried out in companion animal species. Se supplementation above minimum requirements is known to have a huge impact on long term health in other species including humans. These include improved general antioxidant status, immunity, reproduction and a reduction in the incidence of cancer, a primary cause of ill health for dogs (Thrusfield *pers comm.*).

The bio-availability of Se in natural products differs widely ranging from 100% in Brazil nuts to approximately 45% in cereals, around 28% in animal by-products, 15% in mushrooms and 9% in fish. Selenomethionine appears to have a lower bio-availability than selenite, however when selenomethionine is added as a supplement and evaluated separately, the contrary is seen (5.7: 1 for animal tissue and 3.4: 1 for plant based ingredients) in studies from chickens, cats and dogs (Wedekind, Cowell and Combs 1997).

The nature and amount of protein plays an important role in organic Se uptake, by increasing the availability of Se in its selenomethionine form, but does not affect inorganic selenite uptake. Lower protein intakes and feed restriction have also shown to increase uptake. It is claimed that vitamin C increases the potency of dietary Se, improving absorption and utilisation. Based on bio-availability estimates from NRC (1985, 1986), levels of Se approaching the maximum (0.5mg/kg) permitted by EU legislation are actually nearer the optimum for both dogs and cats. For cats this legal maximum is inappropriate, as plasma Se has been found to be up to 5 times that of other animals with no accompanying toxicity reported (Boyer *et al.*, 1978). If the actual optimum is truly around 0.5 mg/kg for both cats and dogs, using a dietary source with a high bio-availability is the most sensible approach. In work conducted using dogs (Lowe *unpublished data*) safe amounts of supplementary dietary Se, when supplied as selenomethionine from Se enriched yeast, would appear to be in excess of 10 times that of sodium selenite.

Bio-availability examined

A calculation based on the background levels of minerals in a typical dry pet food (Table 3) indicates that, in many cases, they provide less than requirement, although it must be accepted that both the total amounts present and their bio-availability are highly variable. Assuming that the supplemental level will be included to meet requirement, bio-availability still needs to be taken into account. The relative proportions of the minerals from each ingredient may be relevant, (e.g. high total Se in tuna) but equally the bio-availability may be low and the presence of mercury (Hg) may reduce the impact of the Se from a toxicity point of view. In this case, inclusion of trace minerals with high bio-availability (which promote body reserves) would be of benefit to ensure adequate supply, e.g. Se enriched yeasts.

Table 3. The total and estimated available levels of trace minerals in a typical dry pet food for dogs for all life stages

	Cu Total (mg/kg)	Cu available (mg/kg)	Zn Total (mg/kg)	Zn available (mg/kg)	Mn Total (mg/kg)	Mn available (mg/kg)	Se Total (mg/kg)	Se available (mg/kg)	Fe Total (mg/kg)	Fe available (mg/kg)
Total	8.1		39.9		19.5		0.16		136.1	
RB		5.85		33.6				0.078		88.0
AB		5-7		12-36		5.0		~0.048		6-13
Req	8.4		140		5.6		0.16		90.0	

Total = estimated total mg weight of mineral in the diet
RB = the mg amount available based on the relative bio-availability of each ingredient to the inorganic source (sulphate etc)
AB = the mg amount available of the mineral in the diet expressed from typical actual availability percentage of the total present
Req = the requirements based on AAFCO which theoretically take into account bio-availability.

It is interesting to note that Se levels of 0.16 mg/kg should be increased to 0.4 or even 0.5 mg/kg to meet requirements based on the likely availability reported by Wedekind et al (1997). Zn levels could be met by the addition of sulphate forms, as the availability is relatively good, however to further enhance the effects of the Zn, it would be prudent to include organic sources, particularly if phytate and/or Ca (which compete with Zn uptake) are present in the diet at significant levels. Problems with such calculations arise because bio-availability is relative, not absolute, making supplementation worthy of careful consideration. Parameters used to measure the relative values also change relative bio-availability (Ammerman, Baker and Lewis 1995) making it important to understand which metabolic process are being targeted, and calculating accordingly when adding the supplemental trace mineral. It is probably wise to consider between 0.4 and 0.6 of the total dietary supplemental transition metal as an organic source. Where permitted, both for physiological and safety benefits, the replacement of sodium selenite with selenomethionine from a selenium enriched yeast would be appropriate.

For physiological responses there are data to indicate potential benefits to increased levels of certain trace minerals, and some of these are confined to organic mineral supplements (Kuhlman *et al* 1998). When trace mineral forms are relatively reactive, such as sulphate, they may cause poor premix stability (Shurson *et al* 1996) and increase damaging oxidative exposure in the intestine (Surai 2002). As a result, the use of highly available sources, such as chelates or proteinates, should be considered in certain diets. There is limited data to indicate that supplementary minerals need not comprise 100% organic forms (Lowe, 1996; Kuhlman *et al* 1998). However the use of organic mineral supplements will more closely achieve optimum levels without excess amounts of total mineral, and avoids problematic inorganic mineral-mineral interactions.

Reflecting the importance of a consistent, bio-available and active mineral supply in animal feed and pet foods, commercial products such as the Bioplex® (Alltech Inc, USA) range of trace mineral proteinates have been developed. The transition elements (zinc, copper, iron, manganese and cobalt) in the Bioplexed minerals, form covalent bonds with small peptides resulting in chelated complexes. Research evidence indicates that these organically bound minerals are, in many circumstances, more bio-active and available than the inorganic forms currently widely used in pet food. Thus, where particular physiological responses are required or marketing strategies are to be adopted, investment in these dietary supplemental mineral sources appear to offer distinct advantages

References

Ammerman, C.B., Baker, D.H. and Lewis, A.J. (1995) *Bioavailability of nutrients for animals* Academic Press, London UK

Boyer, C.I., Andrews, E.J., de Lahunta, A., Bache, C.A, Gutenmann, W.H. and Lisk, D.J. (1978) Accumulation of mercury and selenium in tissues of kttens fed commercial pet food. *Cornell Vet* **68:** 365-374.

Brewer G.J., (1998) Wilson disease and canine copper toxicosis. *Am J Clin Nutr* **67:** 1087S-1090S

Chesters J.K., and Arthur, J.R. (1988) Early biochemical defects caused by dietary trace element deficiencies *Nutr Res Rev* **1:** 39-56

Dyer, I (1969) Mineral Requirements In : *Animal Growth and Nutrition* Eds., E Hofez and I Dyer Lea and Febiger Philadelphia USA.

Fascetti, A.J. and Morris, J.G. (2002) Zinc and Copper Nutriture in the Cat In: *Nutritional Biotechnology in the Feed and Food Industries* Eds: K A Jacques and T.P Lyons Nottingham University Press. UK

Kealy, R.D., Lawler, D.F., Ballam, J.M., Mantz, S.L., Biery D.N., Greeley, E.H., Lust, G., Segree, M., Smith G.K., and Stowe, H.D. (2002) Effects of diet restriction on life span and age-related changes in dogs *JAVMA* **220**: 1315-1320.

Lowe J.A., (1996) An Investigation into the Metabolism of Supplemental Protected Zinc with Reference to the use of Isotopes. In: The Living Gut, *Proceedings of the 12th Annual Alltech Symposium*. Eds: T.P Lyons and K.A. Jacques.

Lowe, J.A. and Wiseman, J. (1997) The Effect of the Source of Dietary Supplemental Zinc on Tissue Copper Concentrations in the Rat *Proc. Brit. Soc. Anim. Sci.* **67**

Lowe, J.A. and Wiseman, J. (1998) A comparison of the Bioavailability of Three dietary zinc sources using four different physiologic parameters in dogs. *J Nutr* **128**: 2809S-2811S

NRC.(1985). *Nutrient Requirements of Dogs*. National Academy of Sciences-National Research Council, Washington, D.C.

NRC.(1986). *Nutrient Requirements of Cats*. National Academy of Sciences-National Research Council, Washington, D.C.

NRC.(2006). *Nutrient Requirements of Dogs and Cats*. National Academy of Sciences-National Research Council, Washington, D.C.

DSM Nutritional Products, formerly Roche Vitamins, (2001) *Vitamin Nutrition Compendium, Optimum Vitamin Nutrition*, Roche Vitamins Inc., Parsippany NY, USA

Shields, R.G. (1998) Vitamin and mineral Nutrition Update. *Pet Food Industry* May-June 4-16

Shurson, J., Salzer, T., Koehler, D (1996) Metal specific amino acid complexes inorganic trace minerals effect on vitamin stability examined *Feedstuffs* **68**: 13-23

Strain, J.J *et al.*, (1999) Optimal Nutrition. *Proceedings of the Nutrition Society* **58**: 395-512.

Surai, P.F. (2000) In: *Proceedings of the 16th Annual Alltech Symposium*. Eds: T.P Lyons and K.A. Jacques.

Tarttelin , M.F. and Ford, H.C. (1994) Dietary Iodine Level and Thyroid Function in the Cat *J Nutr* **124**: 2577S-2578S.

Van Vleet J.F. (1975) Experimentally induced vitamin E- Selenium deficiency in the growing dog *J Am Vet Med Assoc* **166** 769

Wedekind, K. J., Cowell, C., and Combs G.F. (1997) Bioavailability of selenium in petfood ingredients *FASEBJ* **11**: A360

Wedekind, K.J and Lowry S.R. (1998) Are organic zinc sources efficacious in puppies? *J Nutr* **128**: 2593S-2595S

Wedekind K.J., (2000) Selenium in petfoods – is bioavailability an issue? Proceedings of Purina Nutrition Forum (Suppl to Comp Cont Ed Preac) *Vet* **22**:9 A7-22.

Organic mineral absorption: molecular mimicry or modified mobility?

Ronan Power

Introduction

The gastrointestinal tract is one of the first lines of defense against harmful environmental factors, ranging from food-borne pathogens and toxins to several chemical elements, which can cause systemic toxicity if absorbed in significant quantities over time. Aluminum ($Al3+$) belongs in the latter category. It is the most abundant metallic element in nature, comprising almost 8% of the Earth's crust. It is also potentially quite toxic to both animals and humans by mechanisms that are not fully understood (Becaria et al., 2002). Fortunately, the gastrointestinal tract has evolved elegant mechanisms for regulating the ultimate absorption of toxic dietary ions such as aluminum. These mechanisms are highly efficient, as evidenced by recent studies that have shown that absorption of aluminum from the digestive tract is as low as 0.01% of daily intake. However, systems to regulate the uptake of toxic elements such as aluminum have important implications for the systemic absorption of other dietary cations such as ferric ($Fe3+$) and ferrous ($Fe2+$) iron, zinc ($Zn2+$), copper ($Cu2+$), manganese ($Mn2+$) and cobalt ($Co2+$).

Bioavailability

The term 'bioavailability' has been the source of an extraordinary amount of debate, with the result that it is difficult to find a consensus definition of the term. One fairly well-accepted definition, however, was put forward by Ammerman, Baker and Lewis in 1995. They defined bioavailability as "the degree to which an ingested nutrient in a particular source is absorbed in a form that can be utilized in metabolism by an animal". This was elaborated on by Schumann and his co-workers in 1997, who defined bioavailability as "encompassing the sum of impacts that may reduce or promote the metabolic utilization of a nutrient". Finally, in the specific context of mineral bioavailability, most researchers in this area agree with the statement of Dreosti (1993) who wrote: "Physicochemical factors that reduce uptake of mineral nutrients from the intestinal lumen are the predominant influence on mineral bioavailability".

This last statement is particularly important, given that most of what has been written over the last two decades concerning the best means to protect essential trace minerals (thereby enhancing their ultimate absorption) has focused on theoretical transport mechanisms for 'organic minerals' localized at the enterocyte membrane. Although there is virtually no peer-reviewed literature to support such models, they have become accepted dogma in the field of animal nutrition. While such models argue over aspects such as the optimum size of ligand to ensure 'intact transport' of the mineral, they generally ignore the interactions and reactions that occur in the bulk phase of the intestinal lumen and in the intestinal microclimate prior to uptake. Arguably, these events have a much greater impact on the rate and extent of mineral absorption from the gastrointestinal tract than any occurring at the point of uptake into the enterocyte itself. To understand the basis for these differences, it is necessary to take a more in-depth look at the fate of inorganic metal ions in the digestive tract.

Fate of ingested metal ions

Negative interactions between ingested metal ions and certain dietary factors have been well documented over the years. Almost everyone is aware that phytic acid can complex essential trace metals such as zinc, copper, iron and manganese, thereby causing significant decreases in the net absorption of these key elements. Polyphenols, certain sugars and fiber sources have also been implicated as metal binders that hinder the absorption of certain metal ions from the gastrointestinal tract. Of course, antagonisms also occur between trace elements whose electronic structures and states are similar. For example, iron, manganese and cobalt are mutually antagonistic with respect to absorption from the intestine. When dietary iron is low, intestinal transport of manganese and cobalt is enhanced due, presumably, to reduced competition for common handling or uptake mechanisms. However, some of the greatest losses are encountered by certain metal ions which are prone to 'hydroxy-polymerization' reactions.

Ingested metals can be sub-divided into two general categories: those soluble throughout the full pH range of the gastrointestinal tract, e.g. sodium, calcium and magnesium, and those susceptible to the aforementioned hydroxy-polymerization-type reaction. Metals in this latter category are termed 'hydrolytic metals' and include aluminum, manganese, zinc, copper, and iron. They are readily acid-soluble (for example in the monogastric stomach) but upon alkalinization in the small intestine, the water molecules to which they are coordinated rapidly lose protons to form (hydr)oxy-metal species. As the formerly acidic solution approaches neutral pH, further protons are liberated by the water molecules coordinated around the metal in an attempt to maintain equilibrium. This can eventually lead to widespread polymerization of the (hydr)oxy-metal species and, ultimately, precipitation, which renders the metal unavailable for uptake (Figure 1).

Figure 1. Hydroxy-polymerization of hydrolytic metal ions as a function of pH

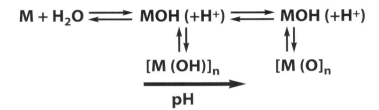

However, these are by no means the only impediments to uptake that ingested metals encounter in the digestive tract. During digestion, luminal nutrients (including non-precipitated hydrolytic metals) are propelled towards the villi of the small intestine but first encounter an unstirred water layer of up to 600 μm functional thickness, and then a mucosally-adherent mucus layer of 50-100 μm thickness before reaching the lipophilic membrane of the enterocyte, where uptake into the body actually occurs and the thickness of which is measured in nanometers rather than micrometers (Figure 2). Thus, it is evident that before an inorganic hydrolytic metal ion can actually be absorbed, it must first avoid hydroxy-polymerization and then penetrate two functional barrier layers that are several orders of magnitude thicker than that of the absorptive cell membrane through which it ultimately passes into the enterocyte. As stated previously, this fact is usually ignored in the literature and attention focused instead on the actual transport mechanisms involved at the brush border surface.

The mucosally-adherent mucus layer

Mucus is produced and secreted mainly by the goblet cells throughout the intestinal mucosa where it acts as a defense barrier and a transport medium (Guth and Engelhardt, 1989). Mucus is made up of large, heavily glycosylated proteins (mucins) that have molecular weights of up to 20 million Daltons. Mucins consist of a protein core with oligosaccharide side chains, O-linked by N-acetyl

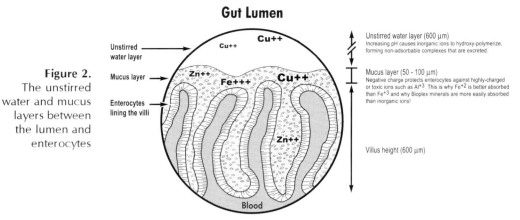

Figure 2.
The unstirred
water and mucus
layers between
the lumen and
enterocytes

Barriers to absorption of highly charged inorganic cations: formation of unabsorbable hydroxy polymers
in ther unstirred water layer and adherence to the negatively charged mucus layer.

galactosamine to serine or threonine. Mucins also contain a high
density of both sulfate groups (sulfated mucins) and carboxylate
groups (sialomucins) that confer an intense negative charge upon
this mucosally-adherent mucus layer. This means, of course, that
the mucus layer has a high affinity and capacity for metal cation
binding and results in trivalent metal ions being bound more strongly
than divalent cations, which in turn are bound more strongly than
monovalent cations, i.e. $M3+ > M2+ > M+$ (where M represents
a metal ion).

Obviously, the ability of metal ions to permeate the mucus layer in
order to undergo absorption will depend to a great extent on their
mobility through this layer. This is inversely proportional to their
strength of binding to the mucus gel and directly proportional to
their rates of ligand exchange. Indeed, the rate of passage of metal
cations through the mucosally-adherent mucus layer follows the
pattern $M+ > M2+ > M3+$. This is exactly why highly charged,
toxic hydrolytic metals such as $Al3+$ are so poorly absorbed. $Al3+$
is so tightly bound by the mucus layer that it rarely manages to
traverse it and is sloughed off into the intestinal lumen and excreted
as the mucus layer turns over. This tight binding of trivalent cations
also explains the extremely poor absorption of ferric iron ($Fe3+$)
relative to ferrous iron ($Fe2+$) (Whitehead et al., 1996).

The unstirred water layer and microclimate pH

As nutrients from the bulk phase of the intestinal lumen move
towards the mucosa they encounter layers of water that are
progressively less mixed. This so-called unstirred water layer is
distinct from the lumen bulk phase and lies just above, and probably

forms an intrinsic part of, the mucosally-adherent mucus layer (Figure 2). Together, they form a pH microclimate that is significantly different from the pH of the lumen and is maintained at a more constant value. Although the exact mechanism by which such tight control of pH is exerted is not clear, it probably involves bicarbonate secretions from the mucosa and/or the entrapment of H+ ions in the mucus layer. Although interspecies differences and variations in the type of electrodes used in study reports make it difficult to define the exact range of microclimate pH values, it is generally accepted that microclimate pH is strictly controlled around pH 7.0 or at very slightly acidic pH values. Because pH affects the charge and solubility of metals and metal-ligand complexes, the intestinal microclimate may have an additional important role to play in the regulation of metal ion uptake from the intestinal tract.

Protected trace minerals

Even a cursory review of the literature concerning the biological functions of essential trace metals, such as iron, copper, manganese and zinc, will make it obvious to the reader why considerable effort has been directed towards increasing bioavailability by protecting them against the adverse environment of the gastrointestinal tract. Early attempts at protecting essential trace elements involved 'chelating' them with ethylenediaminetetraacetic acid (EDTA), which co-ordinates transition metal ions via two nitrogen atoms and four oxygen atoms. These attempts failed miserably, not because EDTA did not protect the metal adequately, but because it over-protected it; failing to release it for systemic use and leading to almost complete excretion from the body.

Chelation chemistry has succeeded in creating a great deal of confusion in the animal feed industry. Today, one hears of metal amino acid complexes, metal amino acid chelates, metal polysaccharide complexes and metal proteinates, yet official definitions remain vague and unhelpful. In real terms, 'complex' is just a generic term to describe the species formed when a metal ion reacts with a ligand. A ligand may be a molecule or ion that contains an atom having a lone pair of electrons capable of being shared with the metal. The metal ion in a complex is bonded to the ligand via donor atoms such as oxygen, nitrogen or sulfur. When ligands bind to the metal ion via two or more donor atoms, structures called heterocyclic rings are formed that contain the metal atom. Such species are called chelates (Greek; chele, a crab's claw) because they resemble the metal atom being held in a pincer-like grasp. It is accepted that the type of bonding involved is co-ordinate covalent bonding and that this can only occur between transition metal ions and suitable ligands (Hynes and Kelly, 1995).

The failure of EDTA as a practical ligand for increasing the bioavailability of metal ions sets important selection criteria for candidate ligands. A good ligand must be able to prevent or interfere with hydroxy-polymerization and perhaps also compete with mucins for metal ion binding. It must not, however, bind the metal ion so tightly as to prevent its uptake or metabolic utilization. There is clear evidence from the literature that amino acids and short peptides are among the best and most practical ligands for protecting transition metals in the digestive tract. When amino acids are used on their own, current terminology designates them as 'metal amino acid chelates'. 'Metal proteinates', on the other hand, utilize a mixture of both single amino acids and short peptides (Figure 3).

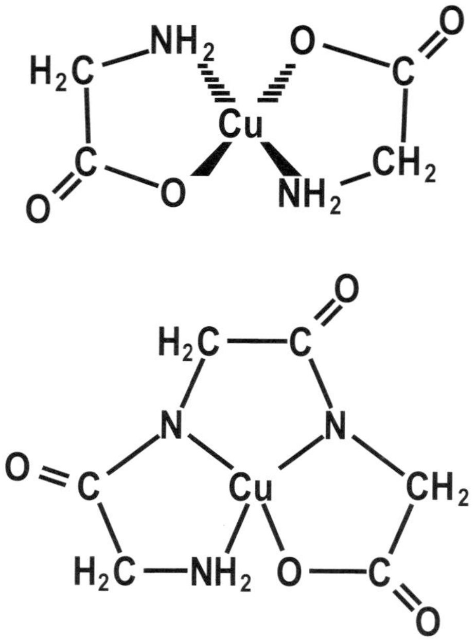

Figure 3. Examples of protected metal ions found in proteinates.

Similar to the debate over the correct definition of the term 'bioavailability', there has been much argument surrounding the optimum size for binding ligands and the resultant metal–ligand complexes. However, the vast majority of such arguments have been based on a finite size constraint for the intact transport of nutrients (and nutrient complexes) across the absorptive enterocyte membrane. From the foregoing descriptions of hydroxy-polymerization, metal-mucin interactions etc., it should be obvious that events occurring prior to metal absorption have the greatest impact on mineral uptake from the gastrointestinal tract, in agreement with the statement of Dreosti. Furthermore, when one considers that the mucins of the digestive tract, which have evolved over the millennia as extremely effective metal binding proteins, have molecular weights ranging from 2 to 20 million Daltons, arguments over the relative merits or demerits of, say, 500 Dalton versus 1,500 Dalton complexes seem rather trivial.

What is important (and should be evident from Figure 3) is that metal ions, protected in the fashion shown, are presented in a reduced charge or electrically neutral form. This has several important implications for the ultimate absorption of the metal in question:

1) By reducing or masking the charge on the hydrolytic metal ion, the ligands prevent or interfere with hydroxy-polymerization, thereby allowing effective presentation of the metal to the mucus layer. Masking the charge on the metal would also prevent negative interactions with dietary factors such as phytate and polyphenols in the bulk phase of the intestinal lumen.

2) The pH of the intestinal microclimate (pH ~ 7.0) favors hydroxy-polymerization of unprotected hydrolytic metal ions. In contrast, these pH values represent the most conducive for tight complex formation between such metal cations, amino acids and short peptides. Thus, the metals arrive at the mucosally-adherent mucus layer in a non-precipitated, maximally protected form.

3) We have seen how the rate of passage of metal ions through the mucus layer follows the order $M+ > M2+ > M3+$. Again, by reducing or masking the positive charge on the metal, the ligand can speed the passage of the metal through the negatively charged mucus layer.

4) Because the protected metal atom does not have to compete with unprotected metal ions for binding sites on mucins, antagonisms such as those commonly observed between, e.g. Cu and Zn, are avoided.

Of course, some of these will be of greater importance than others in assuring the metal's safe arrival at, and ultimate passage through the mucosa. However, all point to the need to question the established dogma that the principal mode of action of organic minerals centers on the exact point of absorption into the body and uses the intended transport system for the ligand (e.g., amino acid or peptide) to smuggle the disguised metal atom across the enterocyte membrane.

Our increasing knowledge of intestinal microclimate topography and chemistry, together with an increasing appreciation of the complexities of mucin-metal ion interactions, make it clear that it is not necessarily an understanding of absorption itself, rather an understanding of the best way to present metals prior to absorption, which represents the key to enhancing the bioavailability of essential trace metals.

References

Ammerman, C.B., D.B. Baker and A.J. Lewis. (1995). In: *Bioavailability of Nutrients for Animals*. Academic Press, New York, pg. 441.

Becaria, A., C. Campbell and S.C. Bondy. (2002). Aluminum as a toxicant. *Toxicology and Industrial Health* **18**: 309-320.

Dreosti, I.E. (1993). Recommended dietary intakes of iron, zinc and other inorganic nutrients and their chemical form and identity. *Nutrition* **9**: 542-545.

Guth, D. and W. Engelhardt. (1989). Is gastrointestinal mucus an ion-selective barrier? In: Symposia *of the Society for Experimental Biology, No. XLIII,* Mucus and Related Topics (E. Chantler and N.A. Ratcliffe, eds). Cambridge Society for Experimental Biology, Cambridge, pg. 117-121.

Hynes, M.J. and M.P. Kelly. (1995). Metal ions, chelates and proteinates. In: *Biotechnology in the Feed Industry, Proceedings of Alltech's 11th Annual Symposium* (T.P. Lyons and K.A. Jacques, eds). Nottingham University Press, UK, pp. 233-248.

Schumann, K., H.G. Classen, M. Hages, R. Prinz-Langenohl, K. Pietrzik and H.K. Biesalki. (1997). Bioavailability of oral vitamins, minerals and trace elements in perspective. *Drug Res.* **47**: 369-380.

Whitehead, M.W., R.P.H. Thompson and J.J. Powell. (1996). Regulation of metal absorption in the gastrointestinal tract. *Gut* **39**: 625-628.

Selenium requirements in cats and dogs

Sarah Todd, David Thomas and Lucy Tucker

Selenium in pet food

The essentiality of selenium and its role in maintaining normal metabolic function is well recognised, and optimum dietary intakes are related to the promotion of longevity and prevention of disease in both humans and animals. However, little is known of the metabolic pathways of selenium in cats and dogs, or what requirements they have for selenium.

Recent investigations into the role of selenium and its optimal inclusion in pet foods have been conducted in a series of trials at Massey University in New Zealand. Along with considerations of level of selenium supplementations, the form of selenium has also been included in this work. Selenium can be supplied as an inorganic form (sodium selenite or selenate) or an organic form (from selenised yeast which provides selenium in the forms found in nature, including selenium-containing amino acids and many other organic selenium compounds). Research in other species suggests that the organic form is more readily absorbed and utilised and does not have the same problems of toxicity as the inorganic compounds.

Analysis of the total selenium content of commercially available cat and dog foods in New Zealand has revealed a wide range of concentrations, and is much higher in canned cat foods compared to any other diets (canned dog food or dry cat and dog food). This is attributed to the inclusion of seafood ingredients, which are known to contain high concentrations of selenium (Table 1).

Table 1.
Levels of selenium determined in different types of pet food

Pet food type	Se level (mg/kg DM)
Canned /moist cat food	1.30
Dry cat food	0.45
Canned /moist dog food	0.40
Dry dog food	0.30

All the pet food samples analysed contained concentrations of selenium above the minimum dietary requirements specified for cats and dogs by the National Research Council (NRC, 1985; 1986) and AAFCO (AAFCO, 2000) (Table 2).

Table 2.
AAFCO and
NRC
recommended
dietary selenium
requirements for
cats and dogs[a]

| | Minimum levels | | | | Maximum levels | |
| | Growth/reproduction | | Maintenance | | | |
	Cats	Dogs	Cats	Dogs	Cats	Dogs
NRC (mg/kg DM[b])	No data	0.11	No data	No data	No data	No data
AAFCO (mg/kg DM[b])	0.10	0.11	0.10	0.11	No data	2.00

[a] Values obtained from (AAFCO, 2000; National Research Council, 1985; 1986)
[b] Dry matter (DM)

These requirements are generally considered to be inadequate, as they are based on extrapolation from other species. They do not account for the varying requirement an animal has at different life stages, nor do they consider the bio-availability of the mineral in its different forms. Mean concentrations of selenium in the pet foods analysed were less than $0.5\,\mu$g Se/g, which are low when compared to the levels necessary for beneficial health effects reportedly observed in humans (Schrauzer, 2002; Whanger, 2004), especially if the bio-availability of selenium in pet foods is as low as previously reported (Wedekind et al., 1997; Wedekind et al., 1998). In contrast, some canned cat foods contained selenium concentrations that were much higher than the suggested safe upper level for dogs (Wedekind et al., 2002) and exceeded the level at which toxic effects occur in livestock (Koller and Exon, 1986). The selenium supplementation required to optimise health in cats and dogs need to be ascertained, and the selenium content of pet foods adjusted accordingly.

Relating intake to utilisation and selenium status

When carrying out research to establish dietary selenium requirements, the response of the animal to various levels of intake must be quantified and the resulting indicators of selenium status of the animal measured in order to determine which levels provide optimum response. Due to the diversity of its functions, various parameters can be used to measure selenium status. These have been well documented in humans and other animals (Ullrey, 1987; Diplock, 1993), however there is no information relevant to companion animals. For unknown reasons, trials in cats showed that GSHPx activities are highly variable, with no clear pattern in response to supplementation (Figure 1).

Animal	Response criteria (mg/kg)	Break-point	Bio-availability	Form of Se supplemented	Recomm-endation (mg Se/ kg DM)
Kittens	Serum GPx	0.12	30%	Sodium selenite	0.4
Kittens	Plasma GPx	0.15	30%	Sodium selenite	0.5
Adult cats	Serum Se Serum GPx RBC GPx	0.10	-	Seleno-methionine	0.1
Puppies	Serum Se	0.06	30%	Sodium selenite	0.2
Puppies	Serum Se (Serum GPx)	0.21 (0.08–0.13)	-	Sodium selenite	Not definitive
Adult dogs	Serum Se, Serum GPx, Erythrocyte GPx	0.13	30%	Seleno-methionine	0.43

Table 3. Estimates of selenium requirements for companion animals (Wedekind et al., 2004)

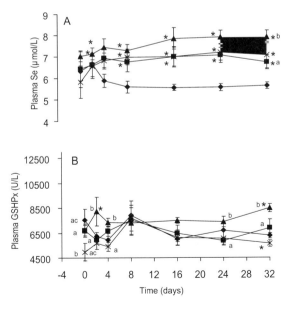

Figure 1. Mean plasma Se concentrations (A) and glutathione peroxidase activities (B) in cats fed diets supplemented with different levels of selenium.

(Control diet containing 0.4 μg Se/g DM (–◆–), or control diet supplemented with organic selenium to give achieve dietary selenium concentrations of 1.0 (–■–), 1.5 (–▲–), and 2.0 (–X–) μg Se/g DM. At each time point: * different from control; values with different letters are different; (p < 0.05)).

Dogs and cats supplemented with both inorganic and organic sources of selenium to a level of 10 μg/g dry matter food, had significantly higher levels of liver selenium stores. There was a numeric trend for those animals receiving selenium in its organic form to have higher stores compared to those fed the inorganic selenium diet (Table 4).

Table 4.
Mean concentrations of liver selenium in cats and dogs after three weeks fed a control diet or a total dietary selenium concentration of 10 μg Se/g

Species	Diet	*Liver Se* *(μg Se/g dry matter)*
Cats	Control	1.4 [a]
	Inorganic	4.2 [b]
	Organic	4.8 [b]
Dogs	Control	1.4 [a]
	Inorganic	7.5 [b]
	Organic	7.9 [b]

Means not sharing a superscript differ significantly ($p < 0.05$)

Dogs and cats fed high levels of selenium (10 μg Se/g dry matter), however, showed no apparent response in plasma GSHPx activities. GSHPx activities were slightly higher in these animals and may be due to higher selenium intake. Whole blood selenium concentrations were variable in cats supplemented with 1.0 to 2.0 μg Se/g DM and there appeared to be a delay in the response of this parameter compared to that of plasma selenium. This is likely to be due to known incorporation of selenium into red blood cells, making them undetectable in plasma (Ullrey, 1987), and whole blood selenium concentrations may be better suited for use as a longer term measure of selenium status as in other species.

Plasma selenium concentrations seem to be a more reliable indicator of immediate selenium supplementation post-ingestion, and reflect dietary selenium intakes rapidly at the supplemented levels of 1.0 to 2.0 μg Se/g DM. Plasma analysis from other cat studies showed increases in selenium concentrations concurrent with increased dietary selenium intake, however these concentrations did not reflect supplementation levels in a linear fashion. Determining any significant relationship between dietary selenium intake and plasma levels requires trials specifically designed for that purpose.

Selenium metabolism

The metabolic response of cats to selenium intake can be determined by measuring the apparent absorption, excretion and retention of the supplement. Excretion of selenium in the faeces and urine of cats confirmed that the proposed role of the kidney in selenium homeostasis (Behne, 1988; Kirchgessner et al., 1997) is also applicable to companion animals. Faecal excretion of selenium, expressed as a proportion of intake, was much greater in cats fed the control diets compared to that excreted in urine. Urinary excretion increased linearly with intake, with organic selenium giving a consistently higher trend in excretion rates compared to inorganic supplementation at levels exceeding $0.4\,\mu$g Se/g, possible as a result of increased absorption.

Figure 2.
Mean concentrations of total selenium (μg Se/kg body weight/day) excreted in the urine of cats after 32 days

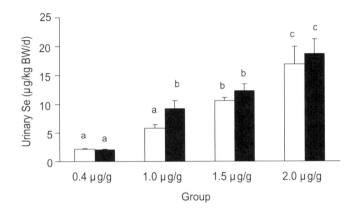

Control diet ($0.4\,\mu$g Se/g DM), or control diet supplemented with inorganic (▢) or organic (■) selenium to give total dietary selenium concentrations of 1.0, 1.5 and $2.0\,\mu$g Se/g DM. Within each form (inorganic or organic), bars with different letters are different (p < 0.05).

Selenium storage, excretion and toxicity

At very high levels of selenium, the capacity of the kidney to excrete selenium diminishes (Kirchgessner et al., 1997) and an alternative excretory pathway is recruited to prevent build-up of the harmful metabolites that may cause toxic effects. This pathway involves methylation of selenium compounds to form dimethylselenol that is excreted by the lungs, and causes an exhaled garlic odour (Shamberger, 1983), which is an indicator of selenium intoxication. There was no evidence of this garlic odour, nor any other physical signs of toxicity in cats and dogs fed selenium at levels up to $10\,\mu$g/g, and it may be assumed that this dietary selenium intake was not toxic. It needs to be borne in mind that the time period in which they received these diets was relatively short, and it is possibly that toxic effects may have developed over a longer period.

In general, apparent absorption of selenium by cats appears to be influenced by the amount of selenium ingested, in the same manner as reported in humans (Whanger, 1998), with higher absorption seen in animals with higher dietary selenium intakes. There was a trend in which cats fed the organic supplement showed higher apparent absorption than those fed the inorganic form, and although there were no clear differences, often as a result of variability within the trial group, this finding was reflected in the amount of selenium retained by these animals. This may be expected, as organic selenium in the form of selenium-enriched yeasts are more bio-available and less toxic than inorganic forms, and have the advantage of being stored and reversibly released during times of selenium deficiency (Rayman, 2004).

There is some evidence to suggest that cats may be able to tolerate higher levels of selenium better than other species (Forrer et al., 1991; Foster et al., 2001) perhaps due to the unique nature of their preferred diet. Although there is little known regarding their turnover of selenium, cats in particular show several peculiarities of metabolism associated with sulphur-containing compounds (Morris, 2002). In a study where high levels of selenium ($10 \, \mu g/g$) were fed, both cats and dogs exhibited the same response, but the degree of magnitude differed between them. Cats had higher plasma selenium concentrations, lower concentrations of selenium in the liver and excreted greater amounts of selenium in faeces and urine compared to dogs. These findings suggest cats may be more efficient at metabolising and excreting higher levels of selenium. Alternatively, the different response of cats to high dietary selenium intakes compared to dogs may be related to the increased requirement of cats for sulphur amino acids (Hendriks, 1999). Further research is needed to investigate these hypotheses, however the data provide additional evidence of species differences in selenium metabolism. This may be another idiosyncrasy to add to the list of unique metabolic characteristics of cats.

Selenium availability and food processing

Special nutritional considerations may arise as a result of the manufacturing processes used in pet food production. Heat treatment of commercial pet foods is primarily used to increase shelf life and achieve a certain physical form (Hendriks et al., 1999), however it can have a negative effect on the nutritive value of the diet (National Research Council, 1986), as heat and pressure can damage certain nutrients.

Trials were conducted using pet food where selenium had been added prior to commercial heat processing, or supplemented directly onto the finished pet food. Preliminary results from a small-scale study in cats suggest that heat processing may affect the bio-availability of selenium (Tables 5 and 6). If a diet contains only a minimum recommended concentration of selenium, reductions in bio-availability may result in the animal effectively receiving an inadequate dietary intake. These findings warrant further investigation into the effect of heat processing on the inclusion of selenium in pet foods and illustrate the need to account for mineral bio-availability when formulating pet foods.

Table 5.
Effect of commercial heat processing on cat plasma selenium concentrations after an 11 day feeding period

Time point	Diet (Se content, dry matter basis)	Plasma Se (µmol/l) mean ± SEM
0 days	Control (0.5 ug/g)	4.5 [a]
	Inorganic (3 ug/g)	5.3 [ab]
	Inorganic + processing (3 ug/g)	5.9 [b]
	Organic unprocessed (3 ug/g)	6.1 [b]
	Organic + processing (3 ug/g)	5.8 [b]
11 days	Control (0.5 ug/g)	4.5 [a]
	Inorganic (3 ug/g)	6.7 [b]
	Inorganic + processing (3 ug/g)	7.1 [b]
	Organic unprocessed (3 ug/g)	7.6 [b]
	Organic + processing (3 ug/g)	7.0 [ab]

Means not sharing a superscript differ significantly ($p < 0.05$)

Table 6.
Selenium excretion, absorption and retention in cats fed processed and unprocessed diets supplemented with inorganic or organic selenium

Treatments[4]	Se excreted in faeces[1] (%)	Se absorbed[1,2] (%)	Se excreted in urine[1] (%)	Se retained[1,3] (%)
Control (0.5 ug/g Se)	100.3 [a]	-0.3 [a]	17.3 [a]	-17.6 [a]
Inorganic (3 ug/g Se)	46.3 [b]	53.7 [b]	55.1 [b]	-1.9 [ab]
Inorganic + processing (3 ug/g Se)	16.7 [c]	83.3 [c]	88.1 [c]	-4.9 [ab]
Organic unprocessed (3 ug/g Se)	38.4 [bc]	61.6 [bc]	80.8 [c]	-19.2 [a]
Organic + processing (3 ug/g Se)	44.1 [b]	55.9 [b]	38.3 [ab]	17.8 [b]

[1] calculated as a percentage of dietary intake
[2] calculated from the difference between dietary intake and faecal excretion
[3] calculated from the difference between dietary intake, faecal and urinary excretion
[4] values represent absorption, excretion or retention of supplemented selenium only (calculated by difference from the amount of selenium in the control diet)
Means not sharing a superscript differ significantly ($p < 0.05$)

Optimising selenium levels

As with other trace elements, it would be expected that the nutritional requirements for selenium occur within a narrow range, outside which adverse (deficiency or toxicity) effects may occur. The lack of associated conditions resulting from potentially unsuitable concentrations of selenium in pet foods tested in these recent trials suggests there is no reason for major concern about the current selenium status of pet foods in New Zealand. However, the previous theory that providing just enough of a nutrient to prevent adverse effects was 'good enough' has been superseded by the increased knowledge of how specific nutrients can optimise health. An animal or human may be provided with the minimum amount of a nutrient enabling it to function without apparent adverse effect, however the full benefits of more suitable dietary inclusion is often not realised. Moreover, there is usually a fine line between benefits and the onset of toxicity. This division needs to be established for each species, different forms of dietary selenium, and the time period over which certain supplementary levels of selenium consumption may cause toxic effects.

The NRC has recently released the revised nutrient requirements for cats and dogs, in which the latest research has been considered and applied. Unfortunately, in the case of selenium, there has been little progress in the determination of requirements in cats and dogs. The work that has been done regarding bio-availability has been incorporated (Wedekind et al., 1998; Wedekind et al., 2003; Wedekind et al., 2004), however much of these data is still extrapolated and are not species specific, thus a complete picture is still not available.

The research carried out in recent trials appears to indicate that, in cats, less than 1.5 μg/g dry matter selenium supplementation in pet food is insufficient to maintain body stores, as indicated by plasma selenium concentrations and tissue retention. There appears to be no additional increase in selenium status when supplementing at levels between 1.5 and 3 μg/g. Providing supplementation at higher levels (10 μg/g) appeared to reverse any benefits in cats by increasing excretion, leading to a negative balance of selenium and consequently, depletion of tissue stores. It seems that a potentially suitable level of selenium supplementation for cats may be around 1.5 μg/g. However, the selenium in these studies was added after processing, and may have a different bio-availability than the same amount that has been exposed to heat processing. In addition, the form of selenium used in pet food should be considered, as organic selenium is retained to a higher degree and is far less toxic than the inorganic form, due to its stability within compounds. More research is needed to confirm these finding in cats and to determine suitable levels of selenium supplementation for dogs.

In summary, results from the current studies have provided an insight into the metabolism of selenium in cats and dogs and contributed fundamental data for future utilisation. More work is needed to further understand selenium metabolism in companion animals in order to determine optimum dietary levels that will convey the health benefits afforded by selenium to other species.

References

AAFCO (2000). *Official Publication of the Association of American Feed Control Officials*. Atlanta, USA, AAFCO Incorporated.

Arthur J.R. and Beckett G.J. (1994). New metabolic roles for selenium. *Proceedings of the Nutrition Society*, **53**: 615-624.

Behne D. (1988). Selenium homeostasis. In: *Selenium in Medicine and Biology*. Walter de Gruyter & Co., Berlin, Germany. Pp 83-91.

Combs G.F. and Combs S.B. (1986). Biochemical functions of selenium. In: *The Role of Selenium in Nutrition*. Academic Press Inc, London. p 205-263.

Diplock A.T. (1993). Indexes of selenium status in human populations. *American Journal of Clinical Nutrition*, **57**: 256S-258S.

Forrer R., Gautschi K. and Lutz H. (1991). Comparative determination of selenium in the serum of various animal species and humans by means of electrothermal atomic absorption spectrometry. *Journal of Trace Elements and Electrolytes in Health and Disease*, **5**: 101-113.

Foster D.J., Thoday K.L., Arthur J.R., Nicol F., Beatty J.A., Svendsen C.K., Labuc R., McConnell M., Sharp M., Thomas J.B. and Beckett G.J. (2001). Selenium status of cats in four regions of the world and comparison with reported incidence of hyperthryoidism in cats in those regions. *American Journal of Veterinary Research*, **62**: 934-937.

Hendriks W.H. (1999). Cats and dogs versus pigs and poultry: a nutritional perspective. *Recent Advances in Animal Nutrition*, University of New England, Armidale, NSW. p 107-114.

Hendriks W.H., Emmens M.M., Trass B. and Pluske J.R. (1999). Heat processing changes the protein quality of canned cat foods as measured with a rat bioassay. *Journal of Animal Science*, **77**(3): 669-676.

Holben D.H. and Smith A.M. (1999). The diverse role of selenium within selenoproteins: a review. *Journal of the American Dietetic Association*, **99**(7): 836-841.

Kirchgessner M., Gabler S. and Windisch W. (1997). Homeostatic adjustments of selenium metabolism and tissue selenium to widely varying selenium supply in ^{75}Se labeled rats. *Journal of Animal Physiology and Animal Nutrition*, **78**: 20-30.

Koller L.D. and Exon J.H. (1986). The two faces of selenium - deficiency and toxicity - are similar in animals and man. *Canadian Journal of Veterinary Research*, **50**: 297-306.

Morris J.G. (2002). Idiosyncratic nutrient requirements of cats appear to be diet-induced evolutionary adaptations. *Nutrition Research Reviews*, **15**(1): 153-168.

National Research Council (1985). *Nutrient Requirements of Dogs*. Washington DC, National Academy Press.

National Research Council (1986). *Nutrient Requirements of Cats*. Washington DC, National Academy Press.

Rayman M.P. (2000). The role of selenium in human health: relevance of selenium status. *Journal of Trace Elements in Medicine and Biology*, **14**: 116-121.

Rayman M.P. (2004). The use of high-selenium yeast to raise selenium status: how does it measure up? *British Journal of Nutrition*, **92**: 557-573.

Schrauzer G.N. (2002). Selenium and human health: the relationship of selenium status to cancer and viral disease. In: *Nutritional Biotechnology in the Feed and Food Industries, Proceedings of Alltech's Eighteenth Annual Symposium*. Lyons TP and Jacques KA (eds), Lexington, Kentucky, Nottingham University Press. p 263-272.

Shamberger R.J. (1983). Toxicity of selenium. In: Frieden E (ed), *Biochemistry of Selenium*. Plenum Press, New York. p 185-206.

Ullrey D.E. (1987). Biochemical and physiological indicators of selenium status in animals. *Journal of Animal Science*, **65**: 1712-1726.

Wedekind K.J., Cowell C. and Combs G.F. (1997). Bio-availability of selenium in petfood ingredients. *Federation Proceedings*, **11**: A360.

Wedekind K.J., Bever R.S. and Combs G.F. (1998). Is selenium addition necessary in petfoods? *Federation Proceedings*, **12**: A823.

Wedekind K.J., Kirk C., Yu S. and Nachreiner R. (2002). Defining the safe lower and upper limits for selenium (Se) in adult dogs. *Federation Proceedings*, **16**(5): A992-A993.

Wedekind K.J., Howard K.A., Backus R.C., Yu S., Morris J.G. and Rogers Q.R. (2003). Determination of the selenium requirement in kittens. *Journal of Animal Physiology and Animal Nutrition*, **87**: 315-323.

Wedekind K.J., Yu S. and Combs G.F. (2004). The selenium requirement of the puppy. *Journal of Animal Physiology and

Animal Nutrition, **88**: 340-347.

Whanger P.D. (1998). Metabolism of selenium in humans. The *Journal of Trace Elements in Experimental Medicine*, **11**: 227-240.

Whanger P.D. (2004). Selenium and its relationship to cancer: an update. *British Journal of Nutrition*, **91**: 11-28.

Antioxidant considerations for companion animal, with special reference to immunity

P. F. Surai

Introduction

Human and animal defence against various diseases depends on the efficacy of the immune system which is responsible for elimination of foreign substances (e.g. parasites, bacteria, moulds, yeast, fungi, viruses and various macromolecules) or the creation of specific inhospitable conditions within the host for a wide range of pathogens. This protective capacity is based on the effective immune system, which is considered to be an important determinant of animal health and well-being. In that sense, a remarkable ability of components of the immune system to distinguish between self and non-self is a great achievement of animal evolution.

It is difficult to avoid nutritional or environmental stresses which are responsible for immunosuppression and increased susceptibility to various diseases. For example, mycotoxins are among major immuno-supressive agents in animal diet. In such situations immuno-modulating properties of certain macro- and micronutrients are important. Research from the last 10 years indicates that selenium is a major immuno-stimulating agent and its' true physiological level exceeds the requirement for growth and development. Its immuno-modulatory effects have been observed in a variety of species when administered in excess of established dietary requirements. Selenium forms an essential component of selenocysteine-containing proteins involved in most aspects of cell biochemistry and immune cell activity. Selenium concentration drops during acute infections compared with the values after the recovery (Sammalkorpi et al., 1988), and deficiency weakens the host immune response, thereby increasing the risk of bacterial and viral infections.

Immune system of animals

There are two major types of immune function: natural and acquired immunity (Figure 1). Natural immunity (the 'innate' system) includes physical barriers (e.g. skin, mucus lining of the gut), specific molecules (e.g. agglutinins, precipitins, acute-phase proteins, lysozyme), phagocytosis (macrophage and heterophil cells), and lysing activity ('natural killer' lymphocytes (NK) cells) (Table 1).

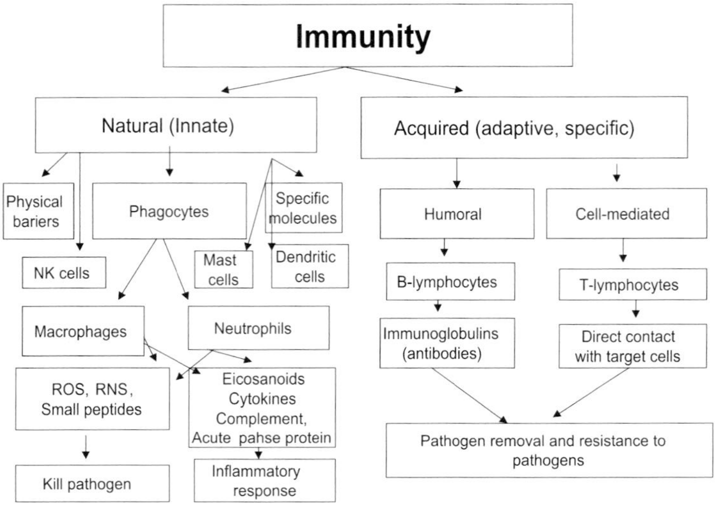

Figure 1.
General scheme
of the immune
system (adapted
from Surai 2002)

Table 1.
Key elements of
the immune
system (adapted
from Kolb, 1996;
Lydyard *et al.*,
2000)

Cells	Significance
Monocytes, macrophages	Phagocytosis, synthesis of interleukins 1,6, 8 and other substances
Neutrophils	Phagocytosis of bacteria, viruses and toxins
Eosinophils	Destruction of parasites
Basophils	Initiation of inflammatory processes
Mast cells	Release of inflammatory mediators
B cells (B lymphocytes)	Production of plasma cells (immunoglobulins = antibodies), antigen-dpecific; 10% of total lymphocytes
T helper cells (Helper T lymphocytes)	Antigen-specific, produce cytokines: IL 2, IL3,IL4, IL5, IL9 and IL10; 55% of total lymphocytes
Cytotoxic T cells (T lymphocytes)	Destruction of tumour cells and virus-Infected cells; antigen-specific, 25% of total lymphocytes
Suppresser T cells (T lymphocytes)	Inhibition of immune reactions (development of autoimmune diseases)
Natural killer cells	Destruction of tumour cells and virus-Infected cells, 10% of total lymphocytes

Cells	Significance
Macromolecules	
Immunoglobulins	Binding of foreign cells and proteins; Promotion of their ingestion by Phagocytes
Interferons (IFN-α; IFN-ß;IFN-γ)	Activation of macrophages (γ-interferon); Inhibition of viral replication
Complement system: a set of over 20 soluble glycoproteins	Destruction of foreign cells
Interleukins	Regulation of specific types of leukocytes
Leucotrienes	Promotion of inflammatory process
Lysozymes	Dissolution of bacterial membranes
Collectines- a group of carbohydrate-binding proteins	Act as opsonins in non-adaptive immune response to pathogen
Acute phase proteins- a group of plasma proteins produced in the liver in response to microbial stimulus	Maximise activation of the complement system

Table 1. Contd.

Macrophages are important immune cells as they perform a range of functions, including phagocytosis of foreign particles, destruction of bacterial or tumour cells, secretion of prostaglandins and cytokines and regulate activity of lymphocytes and other macrophages (Qureshi, 1998). Phagocytosis, the engulfing and destruction of foreign bodies, is the major mechanism by which microbes are removed from the body

Macrophage activation and phagocytosis of foreign particles are regularly accompanied by a so-called 'respiratory burst', where oxidising materials (reactive oxygen or nitrogen species (ROS, RNS)), are deliberately produced to kill pathogenic microbes (Figure 2). Macrophages and other phagocyte cells (leukocytes such as neutrophils, monocytes and eosinophils) can synthesize toxic oxygen metabolites to achieve this (Zhao et al., 1998). In general, the production of ROS and RNS is a characteristic for both mammalian and avian macrophages (Qureshi et al., 1998) and comprise the major metabolites produced by macrophages (Dietert and Golemboski, 1998). Macrophages bind, internalize, and degrade foreign antigens (e.g. bacteria) quickly; it takes 15 minutes for chicken macrophages to kill more than 80% Salmonella (Qureshi et al., 1998).

Natural immunity works rapidly, gives rise to the 'acute inflammatory response' observed in response to challenge by disease. Macrophages also secrete a great number of immune communication molecules, such as cytokines (including the pro-inflammatory interleukin 1 (IL-1) and interleukin 6 (IL-6)), and tumour necrosis factor-α (TNF). They produce cytokine inhibitors, endocrine hormones and neurotransmitters (Klasing, 1998a) which regulate specific immunity, initiating and directing immune systems and inflammation, and amplifying responses, both by communicating with, and presenting parts of pathogens to other immune cells.

Figure 2. Respiratory burst in neutrophils (adapted from Kettle and Winterbourn, 1997; Nordberg and Arner, 2001)

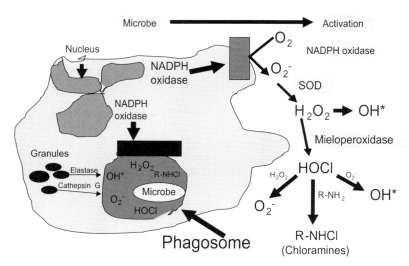

The purpose of immune cells and their metabolites is to destroy invading organisms. Excessive or inappropriate production of these substances can cause mortality. Oxidising materials enhance IL-1, IL-8, and TNF production in response to inflammation, but can also cause harmful effects, including killing host cells, damaging membranes and tissue directly via degradation of essential cellular components (such as membranes), more indirectly by altering the enzyme (protease) balance that normally exists within tissue (Conner and Grisham, 1996) and by causing cell mutations (Weitzman and Stossel, 1981).

Acquired ('specific') immunity includes 'humoral immunity' and 'cell-mediated immunity' (Figure 3). Humoral immunity is mediated by antibodies that are released by B-lymphocytes into the bloodstream. This immunity is based on the production of immunoglobulins (Table 2) which recognise and eliminate antigens by binding and removing invading organisms or toxins.

Table2.
Main immuno-
globulin classes
(adapted from
Lydyard *et al.*,
2000)

Immunoglobulin	Characteristics
IgG1; IgG2; IgG3; IgG4	Largest quantity; provide the bulk of immunity to the most blood borne infectious agents; the only antibody class to cross the placenta to provide humoral immunity to the infant; vaccination asks the immune system to produce IgG specific for a particular antigen
IgA	A first line of defence against microbes entering through mucosal surfaces directly communicating with the environment; synthesised by plasma cells; prevents colonisation of mucosal surfaces by pathogens
IgM	The first antibody produced in an immune response in large quantity
IgD	Present in humans, not documented in animals; functions as an antigen receptor on B cells
IgE	Involved in allergy development and in Immediate hypersensitivity syndromes such as hay fever and asthma

Figure 3.
General scheme
of adaptive
immune system
(adapted from
Field *et al.*, 2001)

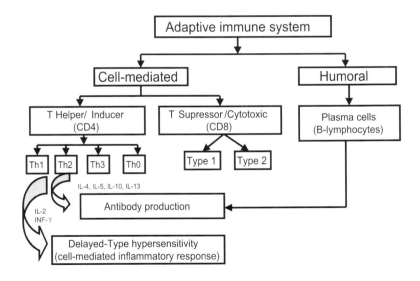

Cell-mediated immunity is based on specific antigen recognition by thymus-derived T-lymphocytes. Cells infected with a foreign agent, e.g. a virus, are detected and destroyed via direct contact between an activated T-cell and its target (the infected cell) (Qureshi *et al.*, 1998). Cell-mediated immunity is responsible for 'delayed-type hypersensitivity' (DTH) reactions, where the body launches an immune attack against an innocuous or beneficial agent such as a foreign graft (Wu and Maydani, 1998).

Interactions between T and B-cells, as well as antigen presenting cells, are responsible for the development of specific immunity. These defence mechanisms are stimulated by exposure to foreign substances and are specific for distinct macromolecules, and increase in magnitude with each successive exposure to a particular macromolecule (Miles and Calder, 1998). In comparison to natural immunity, this type of immunity takes longer to develop, but is highly specific for antigens and has 'memory' in case of future re-infection (Table 3).

Table 3.
Key features of innate and adaptive immunity (adapted from Hansson *et al.*, 2002; Calder, 2001).

	Innate	Adaptive
Appearance in evolution	Primitive organisms	Vertebrates
Induction time	Fast (hours to days)	Slow (days to decades)
Recognizes	Common 'pathogen-associated microbial patterns' (PAMPs)	Unique epitopes on each pathogen/antigen
Cellular components	Phagocytes (macrophages and neutrophils); NK cells; mast cells; dendritic cells	T and B cells
Generation of specificity	Encoded in germline; Has some specificity, no memory	Somatic rearrangement; Highly specific and has memory
Effector Mechanisms	Complement (Alternative pathway); cytokines; chemokines; cell-mediated cytotoxicity	Antibodies; cytotoxic T cells (CTL); classical complement activation; antibody-dependent cell-mediated cytotoxicity; cytokines; chemokines
Soluble mediators	Macrophage-derived cytokines	Lymphocyte-derived cytokines
Characteristic transcription factors	NF-κB (+JNK/AP1)	Jak/STAT, NF-κB, etc.
Physiological Barriers	Skin mucosal membranes Lysosyme Stomach acid Commensal bacteria	Cutaneous and mucosal immune systems Antibodies in mucosal secretions

These two parts of the immune system work together via direct cell contact and interactions involving chemical mediators such as cytokines and chemokines (Figure 4). For correct function, the animal's immune system requires the co-operation of macrophages, B-lymphocytes and T-lymphocytes with various other types of immune cells. Correct response to infection requires cellular proliferation (T-lymphocytes), enhanced protein synthesis (including immunoglobulin synthesis by B-lymphocytes and acute phase protein synthesis by liver) and inflammatory mediator production. Physiological changes resulting from stimulation of the immune system include fever, anorexia and loss of tissue (Grimble, 1997).

Figure 4.
The natural and adaptive immunity interactions (adapted from Calder, 2001)

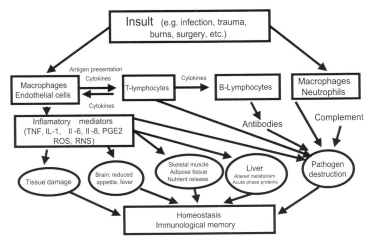

Immuno-modulation and nutrition

Nutrition plays an important role in modulation of the animal's immune system. The majority of scientific literature published on the interaction of nutrition and the immune system examines the effects of deficiencies or excesses of single nutrients (Schoenherr and Jewell, 1997). However, for effective immuno-competence, a balance of nutrients is required.

Energy

Immune response is usually energetically expensive. In healthy adult pets, energy deficiencies are uncommon, indeed up to 40% of the dogs and cats seen by veterinarians in the USA are overweight (Grieshop, 2003). To maintain an effective immune system it is an important task for nutritionists to ensure that energy consumption and expenditure are in balance. Judicious caloric restriction beginning even in adult life, can have a rejuvenating effect on immune response capacity of companion animals (Sheffy and Williams, 1981).

Protein

Protein synthesis is a key attribute of the immune response, making it important to balance dietary protein. Maintaining an adequate supply of essential amino acids is crucial, as an excess of essential amino acids in the diet of companion animals may prove detrimental for immuno-competence. Changes in the immune system have been observed in cats fed a diet containing 5% cysteine with and without dietary taurine (Schuller-Levis et al., 1991). Pathological examination of regional lymph nodes, livers, and spleens showed abnormalities in cats fed cysteine to excess.

Fat and fatty acids

Dietary fat participates in a range of physiological functions including immuno-competence. Whilst fat is an important source of energy, lipids are shown to play a key role as constituents of membranes as well as precursors of active substances such as hormones and eicosanoids.

Certain fats, such as polyunsaturated fatty acids (PUFA), are important for immune cell metabolism. PUFAs consist of two major families: the omega-3 or n-3 and omega-6 or n-6 fatty acids. Their classification (nomenclature) is based on the location of the double bonds in the hydrocarbon chain. If the first double bond is located between C3 and C4 (counting from the methyl end), it is known as the omega-3 (n-3) fatty acid. Likewise, if the first double bond is between C6 and C7, it is called omega-6 (n-6) fatty acid (Ahmed, 1998). Omega-3 and omega-6 fatty acids are not inter-convertible in animals, as the source compounds differ in structure. Feed compounds contain different proportions of these fatty acids, with green leafy vegetables, grass, linseed and rapeseed oils being good sources of n-3 a linoleic acid (LNA) and grains and plant oils such as corn, soya bean and sunflower providing rich sources of n-6 linoleic acid (LA).

Cats require pre-formed long-chain polyunsaturated fatty acids such as arachidonic acid (AA) and docosahexaenoic (DHA) acid in the diet, derived from LA and LNA respectively. Approximately 25% of the fatty acids found in the plasma membranes of immune and inflammatory cells are sourced from AA, and it also forms the precursor of prostaglandins and leukotrienes, which have pro-inflammatory and immuno-regulatory properties (Calder, 1998). Eicosanoids are involved in regulation of major metabolic processes in the body, and functions of immuno-competent organs are dependent on a supply of essential fatty acids. Whether the difference in fatty acid profile translates into improvement of health and productive characteristics is difficult to quantify, and requires further investigation. n-3 PUFA can affect inflammation and immunity by altering lymphocyte, monocyte, macrophage, neutrophil and endothelial cell functions. Such changes in immune system can affect protective efficiency of the body. However, data on n-6/n-3 balance in companion animal nutrition are limited and sometimes controversial. For example, feeding a diet containing an (n-6):(n-3) fatty acid ratio of 5:1 had a positive, rather than an expected negative, effect on the immune responses of both young and geriatric dogs (Kearns et al., 1999). Supplementing dogs with n-3 fatty acids did not affect IL-1, IL-6 or TNF-alpha production, but increased certain prostaglandin production from peritoneal macrophages. Conversely dogs consuming low concentrations of n-3 fatty acids with medium concentrations of vitamin E had the largest delayed-type hypersensitivity (DTH) skin test response (Hall et al.,. 2003).

Lipid oxidation in companion animal diets is a major problem. In a recent study it was shown that oxidized lipids negatively affect growth, antioxidant status, and certain immune functions in dogs. Detrimental effects were evident at 100 ppm aldehyde in the diet, which represents a rather moderate level of oxidative stress. In one experiment, three groups of eight, two-month old Coonhound puppies were pair-fed diets for 16 weeks. The control diet contained < 50 ppm aldehydes, and two treatment diets contained thermally oxidized lipids targeted to deliver 100 ppm aldehydes (medium-oxidation) and 500 ppm aldehydes (high-oxidation). Dogs fed the high-oxidation diet weighed less than those from the medium-oxidation and control groups at the end of the study (Turek et al., 2003). Oxidized lipids reduced serum vitamin E levels, total body fat content, and bone deposition. Furthermore, blood neutrophils and monocytes from dogs fed the high oxidation diet had reduced 'killing' capacity (less superoxide and hydrogen peroxide production) when stimulated compared to the control group, and lymphocyte production was suppressed by dietary oxidized lipid.

Taurine

Taurine has a special role in cat nutrition. This sulphur-amino acid (2-aminoethane sulphonic acid) is synthesised from methionine and cysteine in the presence of vitamin B6, and is found in almost all tissues in mammals. It is the most abundant intracellular amino acid in humans which is not incorporated into proteins. However, cats have limited ability to synthesise taurine and are unable to recycle it via bile salt production unlike other mammals, making it essential in feline diets. Seafood and meat are good sources of taurine which is implicated in numerous biological and physiological functions (Bidri and Choay, 2003; Schuller-Levis and Park, 2003; Lourenco and Camilo, 2002; Degim et al., 2002) including:

- antioxidation
- bile acid conjugation and cholestasis

- xenobiotic detoxification
- modulation of intracellular calcium levels
- participation in retinal development and function
- endocrine/metabolic effects
- osmoregulation, neuro-modulation and stabilisation of the membranes
- modulation of cell proliferation, inflammation and collagenogenesis reproduction by preservation of the motility of the spermatozoa, support of their capacitation, improvement of the chances of success of fertilization and the early embryonic development
- immuno-modulation

Retinal degeneration is a common symptom of taurine deficiency (Hayes et al., 1975), as is compromised reproduction (Sturman et al., 1985; 1986). Taurine physiological levels in cats decrease during certain clinical conditions, e.g. in cats with dilated cardiomyopathy, plasma taurine concentration have been recorded at only 38% of the normal value in healthy subjects (Fox et al., 1993).

Taurine, and its precursor, hypotaurine, are located in the cytosolic compartment of neutrophil cells. The ratio of taurine to hypotaurine is approximately 50:1 (Green et al., 1991). It is considered to be the most abundant free amino acid in certain immune cells (Schuller-Levis and Park, 2003), and comprises more than 50% of the free amino acid pool of lymphocytes (Redmond et al., 1998). The antioxidant function of taurine in macrophages is of great importance (Pasentes-Morales and Cruz, 1985). Hypochlorous acid (HOCl), the major oxidant produced during phagocytosis, reacts with free amino groups ultimately causing loss of important thiol proteins (Carr et al., 2001). Taurine is an efficient scavenger of HOCl, preventing the neuronal damage it causes (Kearns and Dawson, 2000). These findings suggest an important role of oxygen-dependent mechanisms in the cell to maintain an appropriate oxidant-antioxidant balance (Wedi et al., 1999). Depletion of this particular amino acid is potentially deleterious to lung macrophages and pulmonary tissue (Zhang and Lombardini, 1998).

Administration of taurine has been shown to reduce inflammatory bowel disease in rats by increasing defending capacity against oxidative damage (Son et al., 1998) and has been shown to protect guinea pig heart tissue from oxidative stress (Raschke et al., 1995). In rats, the host inflammatory response induced by transplantation of neurons was studied and it was reported that taurine facilitated graft survival (Rivas-Arancibia et al., 2000).

Taurine at normal cell concentrations can inhibit oxidative damage to DNA (Messina and Dawson, 2000). When neutrophils were stimulated with a monoclonal antibody in the presence or absence of the amino acid, apoptosis at 18 h was inhibited and intracellular calcium levels were maintained (Condron et al., 2003). This phenomenon has been observed in human and other cells. (Verzola et al., 2002; Wu et al., 1999; Watson et al., 1996).

Age-related decline in the cat's immune system (Harper et al., 2001) is of great importance, and mechanisms regarding a decrease in total plasma antioxidant capacity of older cats (Harper and Frith, 1999) await further clarification. Experimental infection with feline immunodeficiency virus demonstrated that aged cats developed more severe disease than young adult cats (George et al., 1993).

Vitamin E

Vitamin E is the major antioxidant in biological systems, and the minimum dietary requirement of cats is 30 IU/kg dry matter with diets high in PUFAs requiring up to four times these levels for stability (NRC, 1986). Immuno-modulating properties of this vitamin are well known, however, the results are not always consistent. Following a 12 week feeding trial, dogs consuming low concentrations of vitamin E (17 mg/kg) had lower percentages of CD8+ T cells, compared with dogs consuming medium (101 mg/kg) or high (447 mg/kg) alpha-tocopheryl acetate concentrations (Hall et al., 2003). Dogs consuming low vitamin E diets had higher CD4+ to CD8+ T cell ratios. On day 4 of week 15, the percentage of CD8+ T cells was highest in dogs fed medium concentrations of vitamin E; however, the CD4+ to CD8+ T cell ratio was higher only in dogs fed low concentrations of vitamin E with high concentrations of n-3 fatty acids (Hall et al., 2003). It is interesting that vitamin E alone in doses up to 4.3 IU/g does not improve immune status of cats (Hendriks et al., 2002). However, a mixture of antioxidants including lycopene, ß-carotene, lutein, vitamin E, taurine and ascorbate were shown to improve antibody response to vaccination in cats (Harper et al., 2001). It seems likely that antioxidant compounds, including organic selenium, vitamin E, carotenoids and taurine in combination with other immuno-modulators such as omega-3 fatty acids, could be beneficial in cats.

Vitamin A and carotenoids

Vitamin A plays an important role in immuno-modulation, as it regulates many cellular functions relevant to immuno-competence. Maintenance of epithelial surfaces is an important function of this vitamin, and affects the ability of the immune system to recognise foreign bodies. Impairment of the synthesis of cell surface glycoproteins as a result of vitamin A deficiency is shown to play a crucial role in immunosuppression (West et al., 1991). Glycoproteins are essential components of receptors and are also involved in the regulation of gene expression.

It seems likely that carotenoids have specific immuno-modulating properties. The immuno-modulatory action of lutein has been demonstrated in domestic cats (Kim et al., 2000a). Female Tabby cats (10-month old) were supplemented daily for 12 weeks with 0, 1, 5 or 10 mg lutein, and increased response to vaccination were observed in a dose-dependent manner in Week 6. Compared to control, cats fed lutein also showed enhanced immune cells proliferation. Supplementation increased the percentages of CD4+ and CD21+ lymphocytes at Week 12, and plasma IgG was higher in cats fed 10 mg lutein in Weeks 8 and 12 (Kim et al., 2000a). Similarly, dietary ß-carotene has been shown to increase cell-mediated and humoral immune responses in female Beagles (Chew et al., 2000). Compared with unsupplemented dogs, those fed 20 or 50 mg of ß-carotene had higher CD4+ cell numbers, CD4:CD8 ratio, and plasma IgG concentration. Furthermore, the delayed-type hypersensitivity response to phytohemagglutinin (PHA) and vaccine was heightened in ß-carotene-supplemented dogs. However immune response was impaired in dogs classified as 'low ß-carotene absorbers'. Dietary lutein stimulated immune responses in domestic dogs in a similar fashion (Kim et al., 2000). Female Beagles (17-18-month old) were supplemented daily with 0, 5, 10 or 20 mg lutein for 12 weeks, and results showed that lutein-supplemented dogs had a heightened DTH response to PHA and vaccine by week 6. Furthermore, dietary lutein increased lymphocyte proliferative response to mitogens and increased the percentages of cells expressing CD5, CD4, CD8 and major histocompatibility complex class II molecules. The production of IgG also increased in lutein-fed dogs after the second antigenic challenge. (Kim et al., 2000).

Zinc

Zinc is the second most abundant trace element in mammals and is a component of over 300 enzymes and taking part in:

- antioxidant defence as an integral part of SOD
- hormone secretion
- keratin generation and epithelial tissue integrity
- nucleic acid synthesis

- protein synthesis
- sexual development and spermatogenesis
- immune function

Zinc is required as a catalytic, structural and regulatory ion for enzymes, proteins and transcription factors, and is thus a key trace element in many homeostatic mechanisms of the body, including immune responses. Low zinc bioavailability results in limited immuno-resistance to infection, especially in aging animals (Ferencik and Ebringer, 2003). A variety of *in vivo* and *in vitro* effects of zinc on immune cells depend on its concentration. Important immune cells show decreased function after zinc depletion, e.g. monocyte functions are impaired, whereas in natural killer cells, cytotoxicity is decreased, and in neutrophil granulocytes, phagocytosis is reduced (Ibs and Rink, 2003). Furthermore, the normal functions of T cells are impaired and B cells undergo apoptosis. Impaired immune functions due to zinc deficiency are shown to be reversed by an adequate supplementation. However, high dosages of zinc can have negative effects on immune cells and, as often noted with minerals, show symptoms that are similar to zinc deficiency (Ibs and Rink, 2003). Organic Zn is characterised by improved bio-availability in comparison to inorganic sources and is considered to be better digested, stored and utilised in the body.

Copper

Copper is an essential component of a range of physiologically important metalloenzymes and taking part in:

- antioxidant defence as an integral part of SOD
- cellular respiration
- cardiac function
- bone formation
- carbohydrate and lipid metabolism
- immune function
- connective tissue development
- tissue keratinisation
- myelination of the spinal cord

The immune system requires copper to perform several functions, although little is known about its direct mechanism of action (Percival, 1998). For example, some of the recent data from various studies showed that interleukin 2 is reduced during copper deficiency, as is T cell proliferation. It is important to note that, even during marginal deficiency, immune cell proliferation responses and interleukin concentrations are reduced (Percival, 1998). Copper deficiency is associated with decreased number of neutrophils, along with reduced ability to generate superoxide anions to kill ingested pathogens. In many experiments it has been proven that Cu deficiency lowers antibody production, however cell-mediated immunity is more resistant to Cu deficiency. Copper deficiency appears to reduce production of interferon and tumour necrosis factors by mononuclear immune cells (Spears, 2000).

Inorganic copper has a strong pro-oxidant effect and, if not bound to proteins, can stimulate lipid peroxidation in feed or, even more importantly, in the intestinal tract. Organic copper does not possess these damaging properties, and can be fed to improve the copper status of animals

Iron

Iron has a vital role in many biochemical reactions, taking part in:

- antioxidant defence as an essential component of catalase
- energy and protein metabolism
- haem-respiratory carrier
- oxidation/reduction reactions
- electron transport system

Iron is an important metal required for the proliferation of all cells including those of the immune system. Indeed iron plays an essential role in immuno-surveillance, because of its growth promoting and differentiation-inducing properties for immune cells and its interference with various immune pathways and activities (Weiss, 2002). It is also crucial for the proliferation of tumour cells and micro-organisms, due to its role in mitochondrial respiration and DNA synthesis. As a result, deficiency causes several defects in both the humoral and cellular areas of immunity, one of the most profound being a reduction in peripheral T cells and atrophy of the thymus (Bowlus, 2003). Growing evidence suggests that T cells may regulate iron metabolism, perhaps through interactions with the major histocompatibility complex gene.

Iron is a strong pro-oxidant and, if not chelated to proteins, can stimulate lipid peroxidation. This is especially relevant to the digestive tract where lipid peroxidation can be stimulated causing enterocyte damage, and decreasing absorption of nutrients especially other antioxidants. If iron is included in premix in inorganic form it can stimulate vitamin oxidation during storage. Organic iron supplementation avoids these problems and improves iron reserved in the animal.

Selenium

Selenium is the 'chief executive' of the antioxidant system, involved in a regulation of major antioxidant defences in the body (Surai, 2006). It is proven that Se supplementation improves natural and adaptive immunity in both humans and animals, and companion animals are not an exception to this rule.

Animal feed formulations include supplementation with selenium as a safety margin to prevent deficiency and to maintain good health and high reproductive performance. Reproductive success in all animals depends on antioxidant status, since spermatozoa are rich in polyunsaturated fatty acids which require antioxidant protection. It has been suggested that, during evolution, all animals adapted only to the organic form of selenium (Surai, 2002), as feed ingredients, such as plant materials, contain selenium only in its organic form, which are mainly various seleno-amino acids including selenomethionine. As the digestive system of the animal has adapted to this form of selenium, inorganic selenium (selenite or selenate) is not a natural form for it to utilise, leading to important differences in absorption and metabolism between different forms of selenium. Organic selenium is actively and preferentially absorbed in the intestine as an amino acid, employing similar processes as methionine. In cats, similar to other animals, the absorption of selenomethionine is accelerated by specific amino acid active transport mechanisms in the gut mucosa. By contrast, inorganic selenium is passively absorbed in the gut as a mineral ion. Selenomethionine can build Se reserves in the body (mainly in muscles), but no Se reserves exist in the body when inorganic selenium is fed. Other forms of seleno-amino acids (for example, Se-cysteine) are not a reserve form of the element, hence organic selenium is more effective than inorganic sources, especially under stressed conditions where higher antioxidant demands need to be met.

Se concentration in companion animals' blood serum appears to be substantially higher than that in humans or farm animals (Table 4).

In a recent study with cats, effects of different Se levels were examined, using four treatment diets ranging from 0.95 to 1.03 mg/kg Se (Hedriks et al., 2002). Kittens fed a low-Se diet had significantly reduced plasma Se concentration and GSH-Px activity. They showed compromised thyroid hormone metabolism, where the plasma total thyroid hormones T4 increased and T3 decreased significantly (Yu et al., 2002), effects which can affect thermoregulation, growth and development and ultimately lead to increased mortality in young animals. Se metabolism in cats has some specific features, with concentration in cat's serum being 50-70% higher than that in dogs (Wedekind et al., 2003). Kitten requirement in Se has been recently estimated to be around 0.15 mg Se/kg diet (Table 5; Wedekind et al., 2003).

Table 4.
Reference values of serum selenium concentration in Switzerland, mmol/L (Forrer et al., 1991)

Species	Range
Cat	3.60-10.09
Dog	1.90-4.31
Pig	1.97-3.32
Chicken	1.68-4.28
Humans, 20-60 years	0.78-1.48
Humans, 60-100 years	0.61-1.73
Horse	0.36-1.68
Goat	0.14-1.42
Calves, 3-9 month old	0.19-0.65
Cattle, >9 months old	0.10-0.82
Sheep	0.09-0.54

Table 5.
Response of kittens fed graded levels of sodium selenite(adapted from Wedekind et al., 2003)

Treatment	Dietary Se, mg/kg	GSH-Px, Plasma, U/ml	RBC, GSH-Px, U/10^6 cells	Plasma Se, μM/l	T3, nmol/l
1	0.027	0.31	1.90	0.22	0.73
2	0.073	1.03	3.85	0.99	0.86
3	0.100	1.38	5.23	1.56	0.92
4	0.122	1.72	5.92	2.06	0.91
5	0.210	2.32	5.65	4.12	0.91
6	0.314	2.60	5.81	4.61	1.27

Two scenarios of using selenium in companion animals

Let's consider two different scenarios of antioxidant defence and immuno-modulation in cats and dogs. The first scenario, the most common one, is for animals when inorganic selenium is included in the diet (Figure 5). Under stressed conditions (such as disease or hard physical work), the body responds by mobilising antioxidant reserves in the body and by synthesising additional seleno-proteins. In this scenario the main limitation is inadequate selenium reserves and restricted ability to synthesise additional seleno-proteins, resulting in poor antioxidant protection when overproduction of free radicals occurs as a result of oxidative stress. In such a scenario it would be expected that immunity and health would be compromised and reproductive performance decreased. It is necessary to realise that we are not speaking about dramatic differences, but cumulative or a succession of stresses which can clinically affect animal behaviour and health, especially important in newly born kittens and puppies, as their antioxidant system is immature and depends on maternal antioxidant transfer via colostrum and milk. As inorganic selenium is not transferred to the milk in any considerable amounts, we would not expect an improvement in antioxidant availability through this route in this scenario.

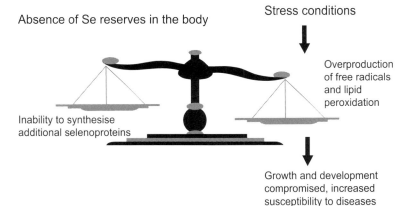

Figure 5.
Inorganic
selenium
scenario

Consider the same case when organic selenium is used in the diet (Figure 6). Benefit is derived from selenium reserves accumulated in the form of selenomethionine in tissue. Under stressed conditions, protein catabolism releases Se allowing synthesis of additional seleno-proteins to prevent damaging effect of free radical overproduction. Adequate storage of antioxidant reserves is especially important, as many stresses are associated with a reduction in food intake, resulting in a reduced supply of anti-oxidants such as vitamin E. Synthesised seleno-proteins prevent lipid peroxidation, and benefiting the animal by maintaining immuno-competence and reproductive capacity. Since selenomethionine is transferred efficiently through colostrum and milk, newly born animals have a ready supply of antioxidants for protection against oxidative stress. Furthermore, seleno-dependent enzymes involved in thyroid hormone activation would ensure correct thermoregulation in very young.

107

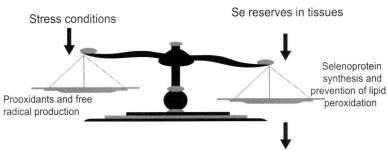

Figure 6.
Organic
selenium
scenario

We need to realise that this scenario has limitations in terms of level of stresses we are considering. For example, when very high levels of oxidising toxins present in the diet or environmental stresses are too high, the body response would not be sufficient to prevent patho-biological changes in the animal. Within the range of everyday stress conditions however, this model/scenario would be effective.

Everyday stresses for pets include:

- **Oxidized Fat In The Diet**. A complete diet for animals contains a range of fat ingredients and some of them are oxidized during feed storage, producing toxic peroxides which further stimulate lipid peroxidation.

- **Mycotoxins** or any other toxic compounds in the feed. It is generally recognised that more than 25% of the world's grain production is contaminated with fungal mycotoxins, making it difficult to avoid them. In many cases they are not readily detectable, but this does not guarantee no contamination. Mycotoxins are considered strong pro-oxidants, responsible for lipid peroxidation. Pet food quality control is typically strict, and tries to ensure only high quality ingredients are used in the diet. However, since environmental pollutants such as heavy metals or mycotoxins are ubiquitous it is almost impossible to completely avoid their presence in raw materials. An analytical survey of 42 elements in 31 commercial canned pet foods was conducted (Furr et al., 1976) found that arsenic, bromine, cadmium, chromium, mercury, selenium were highest in fish-containing cat foods. Lead was consistently high in chicken products. Barium, nickel and tin were also high in some samples. A survey of mutagens (nitrosamines, polychlorinated biphenyls) and toxic elements, as well as the protective constituents zinc, selenium, and vitamin C, from 48 pet foods (Mumma et al.,

1986) found high concentrations of fluoride and iodide in some samples, and high concentrations of mercury and selenium in certain cat foods containing fish. Polychlorinated biphenyls were detected in one cat food.

The occurrence of ochratoxin A (OTA) in canned (26 samples) as well as dry pet foods (17 samples) for cats and dogs has been reported (Razzazi et al., 2001). OTA was detected in 47% of the pet food samples at levels of 0.1-0.8-ng/g. Higher levels of OTA were detected in two pet food samples (3.2 and 13.1 ng/g food). OTA was also detected in 62% of cat kidneys (0.35-1.5 ng/g tissue). When one hundred samples of pet foods including 35 samples of cat food were analysed, low levels of the mycotoxins aflatoxin B1, OA and fumonisins were detected in some of them (Scudamore et al., 1997), and aflatoxin B1 has been reported as being higher in cat food compared to dog food (Sharma and Marquez, 2001). Recently, the fungal profiles of 21 dry pet foods (12 belonging to dogs and 9 to cats) corresponding to 8 commercial brands made in Argentina and imported into Europe were analysed (Bueno et al., 2001). Ten genera of fungi were identified; predominantly *Aspergillus* (62%), Rhizopus (48%), and *Mucor* (38%). The most prevalent were determined to be *Aspergillus flavus,* followed by *Aspergillus niger* and *Aspergillus terreus,* which are all potential sources of mycotoxins. There are also other contaminants in cat's food, e.g. the concentration of bisphenol A ranged from 13 - 136 ng/g in canned cat food (Kang and Kando, 2002).

Mycotoxins are considered to be major immuno-suppressive agents in animals. Using adsorbents to bind mycotoxins and prevent their detrimental effects appears to be an important strategy in immuno-modulation (Surai, 2006). Supplementing with proven products such as Mycosorb™ (Alltech Inc, USA) is an effective means of safeguarding growth, health and reproductive performances in various species.

- **Exercise**. Lack of, or over-exercising increases ROS production and both are physiologically stressful for companion animals

- **Disease challenge**. This one is the most important stress. Immune cells themselves produce free radicals as an important weapon to kill pathogens. Therefore disease challenge substantially increases free radical production and, if not protected adequately, healthy tissues can be damaged. In addition, Se is considered to have a specific role in immune system regulation, which could be independent on its antioxidant functions.

- **Vaccination** is also a substantial stress, and in some cases using vitamin E as a vaccine adjuvant can help by improving vaccination efficiency.

- Various **medications** in the diet. Some can interfere with antioxidant absorption or assimilation
- **Psychological stress**, like lectures, anxious fear

The exposure to potential stresses varies from one animal to another, but overproduction of free radicals and the established need for antioxidant protection are common factors for all of them.

As discussed for selenium, animals have evolved to utilise the organic form of minerals in their diets, and their digestive system has adapted to these forms of Se, Fe, Zn, Cu and Mn. As a result their assimilation from the diet is more efficient compared to inorganic sources.

The beneficial effect of organic selenium for companion animals may be even higher when it is used in combination with other organic minerals; Zn, Cu, Fe and Mn. It is proven that these minerals are more effectively absorbed and metabolised in the body, which could be a major advantage for companion animals.

Antioxidant defences and the anti/pro-oxidant balance in the body are major determinants of many physiological functions in companion animals, and more attention should be paid to this important issue. New forms of trace minerals, in conjunction with stabilised forms of vitamin E available on the market today can substantially improve antioxidant defences, especially in cats, resulting in an improvement in health and wellbeing.

Conclusion

Undoubtedly, the nutritional status of the animal plays an important role in resistance mechanisms against disease-causing organisms, and may influence the outcome of disease in infected animals. When the diet is balanced in major nutrients, the immune response is optimised, however, in many cases, requirements for the antioxidants, vitamin E or selenium, to maintain immuno-competence are much higher than those for optimal growth and development. Protection against the toxic effects of mycotoxins (major dietary immuno-suppressors) by using such adsorbents as Mycosorb® is an important strategy of immuno-modulation. Organic selenium in the form of Sel-Plex® has been proven effective in maintaining antioxidant defences of animals, which are directly related to immuno-competence. Using organic minerals such as Bioplex® copper and iron in the diet of the companion animals is also an important option to prevent negative interactions with other minerals and potential free radical proliferation in the digestive tract. Indeed, immuno-modulation starts from the digestive tract where dietary antioxidants, pro-oxidants and other nutrients interact with each other. The result of such interactions can be positive (improved immuno-competence) or detrimental (immuno-suppression) depending on their balance.

References

Ahmed, J.I. (1998). Omega-3 fatty acids- the key to longevity. *Food Science and technology Today* **12**: 139-146

Bidri, M. and Choay, P. (2003). Taurine: a particular amino acid with multiple functions *Ann. Pharm. Fr.* **61**: 385-391

Bowlus, C.L. (2003). The role of iron in T cell development and autoimmunity. *Autoimmun Rev.* **2**: 73-78

Bueno, D.J., Silva J.O. and Oliver, G. (2001). Mycoflora in commercial pet foods. *J. Food. Prot.* 64: 741-743

Calder, P.C. (1998). Fat chance of immunomodulation. *Immunology Today* **19**: 244-247

Carr, A.C., Hawkins, C.L., Thomas, S.R., Stocker, R. and Frei, B. (2001). Relative reactivities of N-chloramines and hypochlorous acid with human plasma constituents. *Free Radic. Biol. Med.* **30**: 526-536

Chew, B.P., Park, J.S., Wong, T.S., Kim, H.W., Weng, B.B., Byrne K.M., Hayek, M.G. and Reinhart, G.A. (2000). Dietary beta-carotene stimulates cell-mediated and humoral immune response in dogs. *J. Nutr.* **130**: 1910-1913

Condron, C., Neary, P., Toomey, D., Redmond, H.P. and Bouchier-Hayes, D. (2003). Taurine attenuates calcium-dependent, Fas-mediated neutrophil apoptosis. *Shock* **19**: 564-569

Conner, E.M. and Grisham, M.B. (1996). Inflammation, free radicals, and antioxidants. *Nutrition* **12**: 274-277

Degim, Z., Celebi, N., Sayan, H., Babul, A., Erdogan, D. and Take, G. (2002). An investigation on skin wound healing in mice with a taurine-chitosan gel formulation. *Amino Acids* **22**: 187-198

Dietert, R.R. and Golemboski, K.A. (1998). Avian macrophage metabolism. *Poultry Science* **77**: 990-997

Egan, B.M., Chen, G., Kelly, C.J. and Bouchier-Hayes, D.J. (2001). Taurine attenuates LPS-induced rolling and adhesion in rat microcirculation. *J. Surg. Res.* **95**: 85-91

Ferencik, M. and Ebringer, L. (2003). Modulatory effects of selenium and zinc on the immune system. *Folia Microbiol (Praha)* **48**: 417-426

Fox, P.R., Trautwein, E.A., Hayes, K.C., Bond, B.R., Sisson, D.D. and Moise, N.S. (1993). Comparison of taurine, alpha-tocopherol, retinol, selenium, and total triglycerides and cholesterol concentrations in cats with cardiac disease and in healthy cats. *Am. J. Vet. Res.* **54**: 563-569

Furr, A.K., Bache, C.A., Gutenmann, W.H., Pakkala, I.S. and Lisk, D.J. (1976). Element and chlorinated hydrocarbon content of commercial pet foods. *Cornell. Vet.* **66**: 513-527

George, J.W., Pedersen, N.C. and Higgins, J. (1993). The effect of age on the course of experimental feline immunodeficiency virus infection in cats. *AIDS Res. Hum. Retroviruses.* **9**: 897-905

Green, T.R., Fellman, J.H., Eicher, A.L. and Pratt, K.L. (1991). Antioxidant role and subcellular location of hypotaurine and taurine in human neutrophils. *Biochim. Biophys. Acta.* **1073**: 91-97

Grieshop, C.M. (2003). The interaction of nutrition and the immune system: a discussion on the role of energy, protein, and oligosaccharides. In: Nutritional Biotechnology in the Feed and Food Industries. *Proceedings of the Alltech's 19th Annual Symposium* Edited by Lyons, T.P. and Jacques, K.A., Nottingham University Press, Nottingham, UK, pp. 499-507

Grimble, R.F. (1997). Effect of antioxidative vitamins on immune function with clinical applications. *International Journal for Vitamin and Nutrition Research* **67**: 312-320

Hall, J.A., Tooley, K.A., Gradin, J.L., Jewell, D.E. and Wander, R.C. (2003). Effects of dietary n-6 and n-3 fatty acids and vitamin E on the immune response of healthy geriatric dogs. *Am. J. Vet. Res.* **64**: 762-772

Harper, J., Devlin, P., Heaton, P. and Koelsch, S. (2001). Feline immunocompetence and the role of antioxidants. *Waltham Feline Medicine Symposium, TNAVC 2001*, pp. 1-3

Harper, J. and Frith, N. (1999). Total plasma antioxidants in cats: Normal ranges and influence of age. *FASEB J.* **13**: 446.16.

Hayes, K.C., Carey, R.E. and Schmidt, S.Y. (1975). Retinal degeneration associated with taurine deficiency in the cat. *Science* **188**: 949-951

Hendriks, W.H., Wu, Y.B., Shields, R.G., Newcomb, M., Rutherfurd, K.J., Belay, T. and Wilson, J. (2002). Vitamin E requirement of adult cats increases slightly with high dietary intake of polyunsaturated fatty acids. *J. Nutr.* **132** (6 Suppl 2): 1613S-1615S

Ibs, K.H. and Rink, L. (2003). Zinc-altered immune function. *J Nutr.* **133** (5 Suppl 1): 1452S-1456S

Kang, J.H. and Kondo, F. (2002). Determination of bisphenol A in canned pet foods. *Res. Vet. Sci.* **73**: 177-182

Kearns, S. and Dawson, R. Jr. (2000). Cytoprotective effect of taurine against hypochlorous acid toxicity to PC12 cells. *Adv. Exp. Med. Biol.* **483**: 563-570

Kearns, R.J., Hayek, M.G., Turek, J.J., Meydani, M., Burr, J.R.,

Greene, R.J., Marshall, C.A., Adams, S.M., Borgert, R.C. and Reinhart, G.A. (1999). Effect of age, breed and dietary omega-6 (n-6): omega-3 (n-3) fatty acid ration on immune function, eicosanoid production, and lipid peroxidation in young and aged dogs. *Vet. Immunol. Immunopathol.* **69**: 165-183

Kim, H.W., Chew, B.P., Wong, T.S., Park, J.S., Weng, B.B., Byrne, K.M., Hayek, M.G. and Reinhart, G.A. (2000) Dietary lutein stimulates immune response in the canine. *Vet. Immunol. Immunopathol.* **74**: 315-327

Kim, H.W., Chew, B.P., Wong, T.S., Park, J.S., Weng, B.B., Byrne, K.M., Hayek, M.G. and Reinhart, G.A. (2000a). Modulation of humoral and cell-mediated immune responses by dietary lutein in cats. *Vet. Immunol. Immunopathol.* **73**: 331-341

Klasing, K.C. (1998a). Avian macrophages: regulators of local and systemic immune responses. *Poultry Science* **77**: 983-989

Lourenco, R. and Camilo, M.E. (2002). Taurine: a conditionally essential amino acid in humans? An overview in health and disease. *Nutr. Hosp.* 17: 262-270

Messina, S.A. and Dawson, R. Jr. (2000). Attenuation of oxidative damage to DNA by taurine and taurine analogs. *Adv. Exp. Med. Biol.* **483**: 355-367

Miles, E.A. and Calder, P.C. (1998). Modulation of immune function by dietary fatty acids. *Proceedings of the Nutrition Society* **57**: 277-292

Mumma, R.O., K.A. Rashid, K.A., B.S. Shane, B.S., J.M. Scarlett-Kranz, J.M., J.H. Hotchkiss, J.H., Eckerlin, R.H., Maylin, G.A., Lee, C.Y., Rutzke, M. and Gutenmann, W.H. (1986). Toxic and protective constituents in pet foods. *Am. J. Vet. Res.* **47**: 1633-1637

NRC (1986). Nutritional Research Council. The Nutrient Requirements of Cats. Rev. ed. National Academy Press, Washington, DC.

Pasantes-Morales, H. and Cruz, C. (1985). Taurine and hypotaurine inhibit light-induced lipid peroxidation and protect rod outer segment structure. *Brain Res.* **330:** 154-157

Percival, S.S. (1998). Copper and immunity. *Am J Clin Nutr.* 67(5 Suppl):1064S-1068S.

Qureshi, M.A. (1998). Role of macrophages in avian health and disease. *Poultry Science* **77**: 978-982

Qureshi, M.A., Hussain, I. and Heggen, C.L. (1998). Understanding immunology in disease development and control. *Poultry Science* **77**: 1126-1129

Raschke, P., Massoudy, P. and Becker, B.F. (1995). Taurine protects the heart from neutrophil-induced reperfusion injury. *Free Radic. Biol. Med.* **19**: 461-471

Razzazi, E., Bohm, J., Grajewski, J., Szczepaniak, K., Kubber-Heiss, A.J. and Iben, C.H. (2001). Residues of ochratoxin A in pet foods, canine and feline kidneys. *J. Anim. Physiol. Anim. Nutr. (Berl)* **85**: 212-216

Redmond, H.P., Stapleton, P.P., Neary, P. and Bouchier-Hayes, D. (1998). Immunonutrition: the role of taurine. *Nutrition* **14**: 599-604

Rivas-Arancibia, S., Rodriguez, A.I., Zigova, T., Willing, A.E., Brown, W.D., Cahill, D.W. and Sanberg, P.R. (2001). Taurine increases rat survival and reduces striatal damage caused by 3-nitropropionic acid. *Int. J. Neurosci.* **108**: 55-67

Schoenherr, W.D. and Jewell, D.E. (1997). Nutritional modification of inflammatory diseases. *Semin Vet Med Surg (Small Anim)* **12**: 212-222

Schuller-Levis, G.B., Recce, R., Rudelli, R.D. and Sturman, J. (1991). Alterations in the immune system in cats fed diets with excess cystine. *Life Sci.* **48**: 693-701

Schuller-Levis, G.B. and Park, E. (2003). Taurine: new implications for an old amino acid. *FEMS Microbiol. Lett.* **226**: 195-202

Scudamore, K.A., Hetmanski, M.T., Nawaz, S., Naylor, J. and Rainbird, S. (1997). Determination of mycotoxins in pet foods sold for domestic pets and wild birds using linked-column immunoassay clean-up and HPLC. *Food. Addit. Contam.* **14**: 175-86

Sharma, M. and Marquez, C. (2001). Determination of aflatoxins in domestic pet foods (dog and cat) using immunoaffinity column and HPLC. *Anim. Feed Sci. Tech.* **93**: 109-114

Sheffy, B.E. and Williams, A.J. (1981). Nutrition and the aging animal. *Vet Clin North Am Small Anim Pract.* **11**: 669-675

Son, M., Ko, J.I., Kim, W.B., Kang, H.K. and Kim, B.K. (1998). Taurine can ameliorate inflammatory bowel disease in rats. *Adv. Exp. Med. Biol.* **442**: 291-298

Spears, J.W. (2000). Micronutrients and immune function in cattle. *Proc Nutr Soc.* **59**: 587-594

Sturman, J.A., Gargano, A.D., Messing, J.M. and Imaki, H. (1986). Feline maternal taurine deficiency: effect on mother and offspring. *J. Nutr.* **116**: 655-667

Sturman, J.A., Moretz, R.C., French, J.H. and Wisniewski, H.M. (1985). Postnatal taurine deficiency in the kitten results in a persistence of the cerebellar external granule cell layer: correction by taurine feeding. *J. Neurosci. Res.* **13**: 521-528

Surai, P.F. (2006). *Selenium in Nutrition and Health.* Nottingham University Press, Nottingham

Surai, P.F. (2002). *Natural Antioxidants in Avian Nutrition and Reproduction.* Nottingham University Press, Nottingham

Turek, J.J., Watkins, B.A., Schoenlein, I.A., Allen, K.G., Hayek, M.G. and Aldrich, C.G. (2003). Oxidized lipid depresses canine growth, immune function, and bone formation. *J Nutr Biochem.* **14**: 24-31

Verzola, D., Bertolotto, M.B., Villaggio, B., Ottonello, L., Dallegri, F., Frumento, G., Berruti, V., Gandolfo, M.T., Garibotto, G. and Deferran, G. (2002). Taurine prevents apoptosis induced by high ambient glucose in human tubule renal cells. *J. Investig. Med.* **50:** 443-451

Watson, R.W., Redmond, H.P., Wang, J.H. and Bouchier-Hayes, D. (1996). Mechanisms involved in sodium arsenite-induced apoptosis of human neutrophils. *J. Leukoc. Biol.* **60:** 625-632

Wedekind, K.J., Howard, K.A., Backus, R.C., Yu, S., Morris, J.G. and Rogers, Q.R. (2003). Determination of the selenium requirement in kittens. *J Anim Physiol Anim Nutr (Berl)* **87:** 315-323

Wedi, B., Straede, J., Wieland, B. and Kapp, A. (1999). Eosinophil apoptosis is mediated by stimulators of cellular oxidative metabolisms and inhibited by antioxidants: involvement of a thiol-sensitive redox regulation in eosinophil cell death. *Blood* **94:** 2365-2373

Weiss, G. (2002). Iron, infection and anemia—a classical triad. *Wien Klin Wochenschr.* **114:** 357-367

Weitzman, S.A. and Stossel, T.P. (1981). Mutation caused by human phagocytes. *Science* **212:** 546-547

West, C.E., Rombout, J.H., van der Zijpp, A.J. and Sijtsma, S.R. (1991). Vitamin A and immune function. *Proc Nutr Soc.* **50:** 251-262

Wu, D.O. and Meydani, S. N. (1998). Antioxidants and immune function. In: A*ntioxidant status, diet, nutrition, and health*, Edited by Papas, A. M., CRC Press, Boca Raton. pp. 371- 400

Wu, Q.D., Wang, J.H., Fennessy, F., Redmond, H.P., Bouchier-Hayes, D. (1999). Taurine prevents high-glucose-induced human vascular endothelial cell apoptosis. *Am. J. Physiol.* **277** (6 Pt 1): C1229-1238

Yu, S., Howard, K.A., Wedekind, K.J., Morris, J.G. and Rogers, Q.R. (2002). A low-selenium diet increases thyroxine and decreases 3,5,3'triiodothyronine in the plasma of kittens. *J. Anim. Physiol. Anim. Nutr. (Berl)* **86:** 36-41

Zhang, X. and Lombardini, J.B. (1998). Effects of in vivo taurine depletion on induced-chemiluminescence production in macrophages isolated from rat lungs. *Amino Acids* 15: 179-186

Zhao, W., Han, Y., Zhao, B., Hirota, S., Hou, J. and Xin, W. (1998). Effect of carotenoids on the respiratory burst of rat peritoneal macrophages. *Biochimica et Biophysica Acta* **1381:** 77-88

Selenium status and the implications for cancer and long-term health

A. MacPherson

Introduction

Selenium was discovered in 1817 by the Swedish chemist, Berzelius. It followed shortly after the discovery of tellurium, an element in the same series, so named after the Latin, *tellus,* meaning the earth and accounts for his decision to name this new element after the Greek goddess of the moon, *Selene.* The element was originally known for its toxic properties and the noxious smell of its compounds. It was only some 45 years ago that its essentiality was first discovered by Schwarz and Foltz (1957), when they showed that it protected vitamin E-deficient rats from liver necrosis. Since then there has been a rapid increase in selenium research, proving it to be an essential element for humans and animals. Selenium deficiency diseases affecting humans have been recognized, but there is growing evidence to suggest that sub-optimal dietary selenium intakes over protracted periods can result in adverse health effects and that 'supra-nutritional levels of selenium may give additional protection from disease'(Rayman, 2002). Due to its essential nature, the effects of Se deficiency are important in all animal species, including companion animals. Indeed, it can be argued that dietary factors that affect diseases associated with aging are of more relevance to longer-lived dogs and cats, which are usually exposed to the same high oxidative stress environments as humans, than to agricultural species.

The significance of selenium to biological systems can hardly be overstated, for a number of reasons. Its vital role is underscored by the fact that it is the only trace element to be specified in genetic code. It is incorporated as selenocysteine, now recognised as the 21st amino acid, at the active site of a wide range of proteins. It has its own codon and specific biosynthetic and insertion machinery (Gladyshev, 2001). Under specific conditions the UGA codon in mRNA, instead of acting as a stop codon, specifies the insertion of a selenocysteine moiety in protein synthesis, resulting in selenoprotein production. It is thought that up to 100 selenoproteins may exist in mammalian systems (Burk and Hill, 1993) of which some 30 have been identified and, to date, 15 have been purified, thus enabling them to be characterised and their functions elucidated (Table 1). This clearly demonstrates the wide range of their effects and thus underlines the crucial importance of selenium to human and animal health and wellbeing. Evidence as to whether this can be practically achieved will now be presented.

Table 1. Functions of known selenoproteins (after Rayman, 2002)

Selenoprotein	Function
Glutathione peroxidases (GPx1, GPx2, GPx3, GPx4)	Antioxidant enzymes: remove hydrogen peroxide, lipid and phospholipid hydroperoxides (thereby maintaining membrane integrity, modulating eicosanoid synthesis, modifying inflammation and the likelihood of propagation of further oxidative damage to lipids, lipoproteins and DNA)
Iodothyronine deiodinases (3)	Production and regulation of active thyroid hormone
Thioredoxin reductases (3)	Reduction of nucleotides in DNA synthesis; regeneration of antioxidant systems; maintenance of the intracellular redox state, critical for cell viability and proliferation; regulation of gene expression by redox control of binding of transcription factors to DNA)
Selenophosphate synthetase, SPS2	Required for biosynthesis of selenophosphate, the precursor of selenocysteine, and therefore of selenoprotein synthesis
Selenoprotein P	Found in plasma and associated with endothelial cells. Antioxidant and transport functions. Appears to protect endothelial cells against damage from peroxynitrite
Selenoprotein W	Believed to be involved in cardiac and skeletal muscle metabolism[9,10]
15kDa Selenoprotein	Differentially expressed in normal and malignant tissues. Gene located in a region often altered in cancers. High levels in prostate. May protect prostate against development of carcinoma
18kDa Selenoprotein	Important selenoprotein found in kidney and large number of other tissues. Preserved in selenium deficiency
(Sperm) mitochondrial capsule selenoprotein	Form of glutathione peroxidase (GPx4): shields developing sperm cells from oxidative damage and later polymerises into a structural protein required for stability/motility of mature sperm

Selenoprotein	Function
Sperm nuclei GPx	Stabilises condensed chromatin by cross-linking protamine thiols and is thus necessary for sperm maturation and male fertility
DNA-bound spermatid selenoprotein (34kDa)	Glutathione peroxidase-like activity. Found in stomach and in nuclei of spermatoza. May protect developing sperm.

Table 1. Contd.

Dietary selenium intakes and status of the UK population

The first estimate of dietary selenium intakes in the UK was made in 1974 by Thorn et al ((1978), who put the figure at 60μg/d. This was at the same level as the Recommended Dietary Intake (RDA) at that time. In the mid-eighties Barclay & MacPherson (1986) analysed a range of white and wholemeal flours and breads for selenium and using these values reported that dietary selenium intakes had fallen to 43μg/d. These same workers then undertook a MAFF sponsored survey of a wide range of foods purchased regionally across the UK. These showed regional variation in intake of 29-39μg/d, but the mean value of 34μg/d revealed a further marked decline in intake to a level well below the Lower Reference Nutrient Intake of 40μg/d. Other total diet studies conducted around the same time suggested that there had been no decline whatsoever in selenium intake as they reported intakes of 63 and 57μg/d respectively. However the values of Barclay & MacPherson (1986) were vindicated by two further studies, which reported mean intakes of 34 and 33μg/d respectively, proving that intakes of Se had declined by almost 50% over the course of two decades (Table 2).

Table 2. Change in the calculated selenium intakes of the UK population over the past 25 years

	1974	1985	1990	1994	1997
Se intake μg/d	60	43	30	34	33
				63	34
				57	

A real decline of this magnitude in the selenium intake of the population would result in a fall in blood selenium concentrations as has been seen for population groups in Glasgow and Ayrshire, where concentrations were initially at 119μg/l in 1985, but had fallen to around 70μg/l by 1994. In 1985 almost every individual had concentrations above the level which allows for full expression of GPx1 (95ug/l). By 1994 almost none were above this value. Thus there has been a remarkable shift in selenium status in the space of a single decade consequent upon the reported decline in selenium intakes. The principal reason behind this is attributed to the marked reduction in imports of North American wheat for bread-making, from 2, 416 000 tons in 1970 to 205 000 tons in 1995, as this source of wheat contains up 10 times more selenium than UK or northern European grown wheat, which is now the main source of UK bread-making flours. North American soils are alkaline, allowing selenium to exist in the readily available selenate form, whereas in the more acidic European soils selenium is present in the less available selenite form reducing plant uptake. Plasma or serum selenium status has also been shown to be below the level required to optimise glutathione peroxidase (GPx) activity in a wide range of European countries (Rayman, 2000) and recently in the UK in children (Gregory et al., 2000) and in the over sixty fives (Bates et al., 2002), where low concentrations of 71 and 68μg/l were recorded respectively. Other studies have also shown low plasma selenium status (Shortt et al, 1997). It is clear therefore that dietary selenium intakes from food materials sourced in the UK and in much of Europe are below optimal levels. The possible consequences of this for the long-term health of the population are examined below

Immune function

Dietary selenium is known to be important for maintaining a healthy immune response in both humans and animals (Spallholz et al., 1990; Taylor, 1995; Kiremidjian-Schumacher et al., 1994; McKenzie et al., 1998; Turner and Finch, 1991). In deficiency situations, both cell-mediated immunity and B-cell function are adversely affected. The delayed-type hypersensitivity reaction is suppressed in selenium-deficient rats (Kukreja and Khan, 1998), and vaccination of selenium-deficient cattle did not result in effective immunization, reflecting the want of an effective antibody response (Sanders, 1984). Neutrophils from selenium-deficient rats, mice and cattle have low GPx activity and fail to kill ingested *Candida albicans* (Turner and Finch, 1991). Repletion restores the ability to kill. Supplementation with selenium is thought to improve cellular immunity in three ways. Firstly, it up-regulates the expression of the T-cell high affinity interleukin-2 (IL2) receptor thus providing a vehicle for enhanced T-cell responses (Roy et al., 1994). Since the T-cell is a key component in providing B-cell help for antibody synthesis this may explain the stimulatory effects of selenium on antibody production (McKenzie et al., 1998). Age-related decreases in cellular immunity can be partly reversed by selenium supplementation increasing responsiveness to IL2 (Roy et al., 1995). Secondly it prevents oxidative stress-induced damage to immune cells and thirdly, it alters platelet aggregation. Supplementation of patients with 200μg

Se/d effected an 118% increase in cytotoxic-lymphocyte-mediated tumour cytotoxicity and an 82% increase in NK-cell activity over initial values (Kiremidjian-Schumacher *et al.*, 1994).

Figure 1. Relationship between immune cells and their activity (after Jackson *et al.*, 2002)

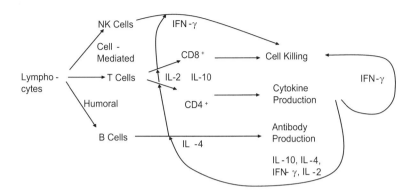

A progressive decline in plasma selenium has been reported in adult respiratory distress syndrome (ARDS) and AIDS patients. It occurs at certain times of HIV infection, and selenium deficiency is now regarded as a classical symptom of the end stage. Baum et al (1997) showed that selenium-deficient patients are twenty times more likely to die from HIV-related causes than those with adequate levels. Low plasma selenium was a significantly greater risk factor for mortality (r = 0.8, p< 0.02) than low helper T-cell count (r = 0.69, p< 0.04). There is an extremely high turnover of CD4 T-cells in AIDS with billions of new cells lost and replaced daily. A sufficient and effective selenium supply is required to keep up with the demand for active lymphocytes (Brown and Arthur, 2001). Rayman (2002) indicated that there are clinical trials in progress with HIV-infected subjects to investigate what effect selenium supplementation has on survival, viral load, CD4 count, immune function and disease progression. Adequate selenium status may protect against HIV progression by maintaining host immune competence and appropriate redox control.

Immune system cells may also have an important functional requirement for selenium. Activated T-cells exhibit an enhanced selenophosphate synthetase (SPS2) activity (Guimaraes *et al.*, 1996) for the synthesis of selenocysteine, the essential amino acid for selenoproteins thus showing their importance to activated T-cell function and the control of the immune response. Taylor (1999) has shown that the mRNA's of several genes associated with T-cells (e.g. IL2 receptor α-subunit, CD4) are theoretically able to encode functional selenoproteins which suggests that selenium's role in immune function may be greater than previously suspected.

Viral Infections

Beck and her research team (1995) demonstrated that when selenium-deficient mice were inoculated with a benign strain of coxsackie virus (CVB3/0), it became virulent and caused myocarditis with similarities to human symptoms of the disease. This was found to be associated with six separate point mutations in the viral genome. When the altered virus was recovered from these mice and inoculated into selenium-adequate mice it still caused heart damage, indicating that the mutation was irreversible. Keshan disease occurs in selenium-deficient parts of China and the presence of coxsackie virus may be a co-factor in the occurrence of the cardiomyopathy that affects these patients – primarily young women and girls. More recently Beck et al. (2001) have shown that selenium-deficient mice infected with a mild strain of influenza virus (Influenza A/Bangkok/1/79) go on to develop a much more severe and prolonged lung inflammation than selenium-adequate mice. As for the coxsackie virus, passage through selenium-deficient animals produced 29 nucleotide changes in the gene for the internal viral M1 matrix protein which was previously believed to be relatively stable. Beck believes that the changes in both viruses involve an oxidative stress mechanism.

Selenium deficiency, through its effect on the genome of RNA viruses, can contribute to the appearance of new viral strains. Other RNA viruses potentially susceptible to mutations resulting in increased virulence include HIV, Ebola, common cold, polio and hepatitis. Selenium also affords protection against hepatitis B and C and against the progression of the disease to liver cancer (Yu *et al.*, 1997; 1999). A recent study by Jackson et al (2002) in the UK, using selenium-supplemented subjects, found an increase in cell-mediated immunity which was accompanied by more rapid clearance of live attenuated polio virus, supporting the findings of Beck and her colleagues.

On the downside there is evidence to suggest that viruses themselves incorporate selenium into viral selenoproteins thus lowering the host's ability to mount an effective immune response. Several viruses (molluscum contagiosum, HIV-1 and 2, coxsackie virus B3, hepatitis B and C, Ebola and the measles virus) contain sequences similar to GPx.

Reproduction

Selenium has long been recognised in animal husbandry as being essential for successful reproduction (Hartley, 1963; Wilkins and

Kilgour, 1982). Miscarriage with no apparent cause has been shown to be associated with Se deficiency (Stuart and Oehme, 1982) while supplementation with selenium prevented early pregnancy loss in sheep (Hidiroglou, 1979).

Se is essential for male fertility, being required for testosterone biosynthesis and the formation and normal maturation and development of spermatozoa (Behne et al., 1996; Pfeifer et al., 2001). In rat's testis, selenium concentration rises markedly at puberty with the spermatozoa having by far the highest level of all compartments (Behne et al., 1986). Selenium-depleted rats produced sperm with impaired motility and anomalies in the mid-piece (Wu, et al., 1979). Malformations of the sperm head have been observed in selenium-deficient mice (Watanabe and Endo, 1991), while testicular atrophy and complete disruption of spermatogenesis has been recorded in severely selenium-depleted rats (Behne et al., 1996). Selenium, in its 34kD selenoprotein form, is found only in the testis and spermatozoa, and has been identified as a specific sperm nuclei glutathione peroxidase (snGPx) with properties similar to phospholipid hydroperoxide glutathione peroxidase. In rats snGPx is expressed in the nuclei of the late spermatids where it is the only selenoprotein present. Its appearance coincides with the reorganisation of DNA, which leads to highly condensed chromatin, stabilised by cross-linked protamine thiols. In selenium-depleted rats with only one third of the normal snGPx concentration chromatin condensation was severely disturbed. It appears that snGPx acts as a protamine thiol peroxidase responsible for disulphide cross-linking by reduction of reactive oxygen species. Its dual function in chromatin condensation and the protection of sperm DNA against oxidation is necessary to ensure sperm quality and male fertility. Se concentration in seminal plasma correlated positively with sperm count ($R^2 = 0.15$, $p > 0.001$) and total sperm concentration ($R^2 = 0.21$, $p > 0.001$) in a group of sub-fertile Norwegian men (Oldereid et al., 1998). An explanation for these findings has recently been afforded by the work of Ursini and colleagues (1999). They found that a form of glutathione peroxidase (GPx4), believed to shield developing sperm cells from oxidative damage, polymerises in mature sperm into a structural protein in the mitochondrial capsule of the mid-piece region. As GPx4 accounts for about 50% of the capsule material, it seems likely that it is this polymerisation that confers the structural integrity required for sperm stability and motility.

Support for this interpretation came from studies at Glasgow Royal Infirmary, in which supplementation of sub-fertile men with 100μg selenium per day for three months significantly increased sperm motility (p = 0.023) (Scott et al, 1998) Eleven percent of men receiving the active supplement achieved paternity as compared to none in the placebo group. However administration of double this quantity of selenium to sub fertile Polish men over a similar period, showed no beneficial effect on sperm motility (Iwanier and Zachara, 1995).

Barrington and colleagues found significantly lower serum Se in women who suffered either first-trimester (p = 0.0054) or recurrent miscarriages (p = 0.014) (Barrington *et al.*, 1996; 1997). He suggests that early pregnancy loss may be linked to reduced antioxidant protection of biological membranes and DNA by relatively low levels of the Se-dependent GPx. A subsequent study found lower Se levels in non-pregnant women suffering recurrent miscarriage than in controls, but the difference did not reach significance (Nicoll *et al.*, 1999). However, the choice of control group can be criticised in this study, as it did not exclude women who had suffered a miscarriage.

Infertility affects around 1 in 7 couples and a diagnosis of sperm dysfunction is made in approximately one third of cases (Templeton, 1995). Spermatozoal dysfunction is the single most common cause of infertility (Kessopoulou *et al.*, 1995). There is growing evidence that reactive oxygen species are involved in the peroxidative damage of human spermatozoa seen in many cases of male infertility. These effects are thought to be counteracted by a number of antioxidant systems which semen is thought to possess. Glutathione peroxidase has been assumed to play a role in protecting cells from harmful effects of toxic metabolites and free radicals by preventing lipid peroxidation of membranes. Selenium constitutes an essential component of this system and has both structural and enzymatic roles, the latter context being best known as an antioxidant and catalyst for the production of thyroid hormone. A positive correlation has been observed between selenium and zinc in seminal plasma and sperm density in normospermic men but not in oligospermic men (Xu *et al.*, 1993) and sperm morphology (Noack-Fuller *et al.*, 1993). Other studies have however shown that although selenium supplementation enhances the element in seminal fluid, it does not change the spermatozoal quality characteristics in sub-fertile men (Iwanier and Zachara, 1995).

Cancer

Exposure to the modern environment, cigarette smoke, and indoor living are all thought to contribute to the physiological stresses that can increase DNA damage, causing cancer, This is true for the pets which live alongside humans as much as for the humans themselves. Much evidence exists to suggest that selenium affords protection against some forms of cancer and that higher intakes are associated with reduced cancer risk. Supplementation with selenium resulted in a reduced incidence of tumours from carcinogenic chemicals or viruses in two thirds of reported studies with experimental animals (Coombs and Lu, 2001). Many epidemiological studies have revealed an inverse relationship between cancer mortality and selenium intake (Coombs and Gray, 1998). Prospective studies with up to 11,000 human subjects have shown low selenium status to be associated with an increased risk (from two to six fold higher) of cancer incidence or mortality (Kok et al., 1987), with a Finnish study reporting reduced risk of stomach, pancreas and lung cancer in Se-adequate men.

In Taiwan a study with 7,342 men revealed a significant inverse relationship between selenium concentrations in stored plasma and the later development of hepatocellular carcinoma (HCC). These men had chronic hepatitis virus B or C infection, which is a well-known risk factor for HCC (Wu et al., 1999). Selenium appears to protect the individual against progression of the disease to liver cancer. In a prospective study involving 34,000 men in the USA, those with low toenail selenium concentrations were at three times the risk of developing advanced prostate cancer compared to those with the highest (Yoshizawa et al., 1998). In a case-control study on men from Baltimore low plasma selenium was associated with a four to five fold increased risk of developing prostate cancer (Brooks et al., 2001).

Not many studies have yet been undertaken which have examined the effect of supplementation with selenium as a single agent on cancer prevention. In the NPC (National Prevention of Cancer) trial an investigation of 1,312 people with a history of non-melanoma skin cancer were randomly given either a placebo or 200μg selenium/day as selenium-enriched yeast. Although there was no effect on the development of skin cancer, selenium supplementation did cause a 50% reduction in overall mortality from this cancer, and resulted in a 37% decline in total cancer incidence with 63, 58 and 46% fewer prostate, colon and lung cancers respectively. The strongest treatment effect was found in subjects with the lowest plasma selenium concentrations (< 106μgSe/l) Clark et al., 1996). Further analysis of the data at the conclusion of the trial showed that there was a significant reduction in lung cancer incidence only among subjects with low baseline selenium concentrations (Reid et al., 2002). The final results of the trial did not confirm the effect on colorectal cancer (Duffield-Lillico et al., 2002).

Other intervention trials have been conducted in China where HCC is the third highest cause of cancer mortality. In Qidong county,

15% of adults carry the Hepatitis B surface antigen which renders them 200 times more likely to develop HCC. When 226 carriers were randomly given 200µg selenium as selenium-enriched yeast or placebo, no cases of HCC occurred in the treatment group after 4 years while 7 subjects in the placebo group had developed HCC (Yu *et al.*, 1999). In a separate study by the same researchers, salt fortified with selenium reduced the incidence of HCC in a Chinese township by 35% over a 6 year period compared to control townships.

Many of the responses to selenium reported have been as a result of supranutritional intakes of the element. Animal studies have shown repeatedly that selenium intakes in excess of requirements can inhibit tumourigenesis (Coombs, 1989; El-Bayoumy, 1991). The NPC trial results showed that selenium supplementation of non-deficient subjects effectively reduced cancer risk.

Studies in China recorded reductions in the risk of liver and oesophogeal cancers following selenium supplementation (Blot *et al.*, 1993). Coombs (2001) states that it is now widely accepted that high level exposure to at least some selenium compounds can be anti-tumourigenic. The anti-tumourigenic effect in experimental models has involved the use of selenium intakes of around 100µg/kg body weight whereas the selenoproteins only require 0.5µgSe/kg body weight for maximum expression. Consequently it has been concluded that the anti-carcinogenic effects of high selenium intakes are due to the production of selenium metabolites such as methylselenol (Ganther, 1999; Ip *et al.*, 2001). Se enhances carcinogen metabolism, affects gene expression, improves immune surveillance, alters cell cycling, promotes apoptosis and inhibits neo-angiogenesis. Some workers suggest that it would be premature to rule out selenoproteins from all roles in cancer prevention, as they may exhibit different expression patterns at high concentration or where genetic or environmental stresses are involved, although the functions of many have yet to be determined (Gladyshev *et al.*, 2001).GPx2 may be involved in preventing colon cancer and the 15kDa selenoprotein may protect against prostate cancer (Wingler *et al.*, 1999; 2000).

Selenium intakes

The daily dietary intakes of selenium in various European countries are given in Table 3, and illustrate that intakes in most European countries are below the RNI of 75 and 60µg/d for adult men and women respectively. The exceptions are Greece, Switzerland, Finland and parts of Russia. In Finland the adequate intakes are due to the practice of adding selenium to all fertilizers since 1984 as prior to this, Finnish intakes were amongst the lowest in the world.

Importation of North American wheat helps to maintain the level of intakes in Switzerland, while both Greece and large parts of Russia have higher indigenous soil selenium concentrations. Two belts of low selenium areas pass through Europe – from north to south (Scandinavia to the Balkans) and from east to west (Belorussia to France). The Czech Republic lies at the crossing of these belts and there are indications of serious deficiency in that country (Kvicala and Kroupova, 1999). Anke et al (2002) have stated that the flora grown on neutral soils in Central Europe are selenium-rich, but those grown on acidic soils formed by weathering of slate, granite, as well as alluvial soils bear a selenium-poor vegetation. As indicated earlier the bioavailability of soil selenium increases significantly with pH.

Table 3.
The reported adult intake of selenium in various European countries

Country	Se intake (μg/d)	Year
Austria	48	1998
Belgium	45	1994
Croatia	27	1998
Czech Republic	15-22	2000
Denmark	40	1998
England	34-39	1995-9
Finland	25	1984
	67-110	1995-6
France	29-43	1994-7
Germany	35-42	1993-5
Greece	110	1990
Hungary	41-92	1992
Italy	49	1991
Netherlands	67	1993
Poland	11-94	1995-9
Portugal	37 (10-100)	1990
Russia	54-80	1994-8
Scotland	32	1995
Serbia	30	1995
Slovakia	27-43	1998
Spain	60	1991
Sweden	38	2000
Switzerland	70	1993
Turkey	32	1991

Selenium concentrations in European wheat

There appears to have been some increase in the selenium content of Swiss wheat since the first half of last century when the median concentration recorded was only 11μg/kg as compared to 23μg/kg in 1996. In the UK in contrast there was no change in the mean concentration (25μg/kg) recorded over the admittedly shorter period from 1982 to 1998.

Country	Se concentration (μg/kg)	Year
Austria	2-160	2000
Russia	100-200	1999
	46-577	
Russia (low Se areas)	34-60	1997
Ukraine	64-74	1997
Switzerland	23* (2-525)	1996
(archived samples)	11* (0.5-415)	1920-1950
Norway	16	2001
Spain	28	2000
United Kingdom	25	1982
	33	1992
	25	1998
Sweden	2-16	2000
Germany	69 (13-130)	2000
Czech Republic	25 (5-154)	1992

*median value

A survey of the selenium content of UK flours obtained from mills across the country and undertaken in 1997 revealed 75% were < 50μg/kg with only 10% > 100μg/kg and this despite the fact that 54% had protein contents > 12%. Selenium content of flour has previously been shown to be directly related to its protein concentration (Barclay and MacPherson, 1986). Table 5 presents the summarised data from the survey.

Table 5.
Selenium
concentrations
(mean and range
μg/kg DM) of
flour samples
from UK mills

Source	No. of samples	Mean Se concentration	Range	% < 50μg/kg
Hull	10	56.3	29-144	60
Rotherham	21	38.8	19-65	86
Manchester	15	113.6	25-463	53
Glasgow	3	22.3	15-32	100
Felixstowe	3	54.0	45-68	67
Barry	16	39.1	20-72	94
Kirkcaldy	12	127.9	24-476	67
Silloth	3	94	38-139	33

The data presented in Tables 3-5 show that selenium intakes in many European countries fail to meet the recommended intakes of the element (UKRNI 75μg/d for men; 60μg/d for women) and that in many cases they do not even provide the lower reference intake of 40μg/d which only allows for some two thirds of the full expression of the selenoenzymes. The generally low level of selenium in European wheats and the high proportion of UK flours with < 50μgSe/kg suggest that any diets based on these would require to be supplemented to ensure an adequate level of intake. Rayman (2002) has recently reviewed a range of strategies to achieve higher selenium intakes. Food fortification is also possible, and practices such as adding Se to bread-making flour could raise human dietary intakes significantly. High selenium pork is produced in Korea (Cole, 2000) while selenium-enriched eggs (Surai et al., 2000) and lamb (Molnar et al., 1997) have been developed in Scotland. Apparently Marks and Spencer has developed a range of foods which include 50μg selenium per serving. Coombs (2001) lists several vegetables that have been enriched with selenium including broccoli, brussels sprouts, onions, celery, mushrooms, mussels and beverages including tea and beer. The brassicas naturally have high concentrations of S-containing amino acids and these have the greatest potential for accumulating selenium. The element is best supplied in organic forms (Figure 2) as this leads to higher tissue selenium levels. This is because the organic forms can be synthesised non-specifically into the body protein, forming storage reserves.

The form of selenium present in foodstuffs varies. In selenium-enriched yeast, the dominant form is selenomethionine while in selenium-enriched garlic it is gamma-glutamyl-Se-methylseleno-cysteine (Korhola et al., 1986). Selenium-enriched yeast was used in the National Prevention of Cancer trial, where it was found to be effective in reducing cancer risk. Selenomethionine comprises around 65% of the selenium in selenium-enriched yeast, the remainder includes selenocysteine, and both are metabolised to the potentially anti-carcinogenic H_2Se form, as well as to a smaller amount of seleno-methylselenocysteine, a precursor of another putative anti-carcinogenic metabolite methylselenol (Ip et al., 1990). On the basis of a trial with rats it has been concluded that selenium from selenium yeast was more bioavailable than inorganic selenite forms (Yoshida et al., 1999). In a selenium supplementation study of young children in China selenite and selenium-yeast were equally effective in raising GPx activity in plasma, red blood cells and platelets but the selenium yeast had a longer lasting effect on maintaining the body pool of selenium and may therefore be the better prophylactic treatment for Keshan Disease. The selenium from high selenium broccoli has been shown to protect rats against colorectal cancer (Finley et al., 2000). It has been suggested that the close similarity of selenised yeast to the natural forms of selenium found in crops, plus the careful control that can be exercised of the selenium content in yeast production, make it a useful and environmentally safe supplement for use with livestock (Lyons and

Oldfield, 1996). Selenium from animal sources is apparently bound in an unavailable chemical form and is not incorporated into blood proteins as readily as selenium supplied as organic supplements (Bugel *et al.*, 2002).

Figure 2.
Organic and
inorganic forms
of selenium

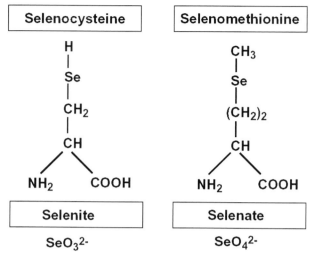

MacPherson (1987) found that a single injection with a barium selenate preparation (*Deposel*) increased deficient plasma selenium levels to normal and successfully maintained them for a year in adult cattle and 18 months in ewes. Selenomethionine was more efficient than inorganic selenium in raising muscle, but not organ, selenium concentrations in sheep (Molnar *et al.*, 1997). Similar results were reported for pigs where organic selenium increased selenium levels more effectively than inorganic in loin, liver and pancreas (Mahan *et al.*, 1999). With younger pigs, however, organic selenium supplementation led to much higher increases in liver, loin, lung and kidney selenium concentrations than those following inorganic supplementation (Kim and Mahan, 2001). Ortman and Pehrson (1997) reported that selenium yeast gave a greater boost to bovine plasma selenium than either selenite or selenate selenium and gave an even greater increase to milk selenium in contrast to almost no response to inorganic supplementation.

Conclusion

This paper has reviewed the health effects associated with inadequate dietary intakes of selenium in humans and animals, which have especial relevance for longer lived species, such as humans and companion animals which are exposed to oxidising stressors in their environment, and are more likely to suffer from cancers and other degenerative diseases associated with aging.

Low Se status risks include lowered immune function and increased susceptibility to disease and an enhanced probability of disease progression. Evidence for a link between selenium deficiency and the virulence of viral infections has been investigated, and its involvement, through its effect on the genome, in the emergence of new viral strains is important for human health on a global scale. Se deficiency has also been related to an increased risk of certain forms of cancer, and linked to both male and female infertility, where it is vital for sperm maturation and motility and to prevent early miscarriage. Adequate Se is involved with preventing many other chronic diseases, such as cardiovascular disease, iodine deficiency disorders, chondrodystrophies and asthma outside the scope of this review. It is clearly important therefore that the selenium status of individuals and populations is kept at a sufficiently high level to minimise these possible adverse consequences.

Dietary intakes from food prepared using raw materials sourced in the UK and in many other European countries have been revealed as being below the RNI, and in some instances below the LRNI. Diets based on these, either for humans or in the context of this publication, their pets would require supplementation with a suitably available source of Se to ensure adequate intake. It would appear that such supplementation would be most effective if offered as organic (e.g. selenium yeast) rather than inorganic form.

References

Adams, M.L., Lombi, E., Zhao, F.J. and McGrath, S.P. (2002) Evidence of low selenium concentrations in UK bread-making wheat grain. *J. Sci. Fd. Agric.* **82,** 1160 1165.

Alfthan, G., Bogye, G., Aro, A. and Feher, J. (1992) The human selenium status in Hungary. *J. Trace. Elem. Electrol. Health Dis.* **68,** 233-238.

Allan, C.B., Lacourciere, G.M. and Stadtman, T.C. (1999) Responsiveness of selenoproteins to dietary selenium. *Annual Review of Nutrition,* **19,** 1-16.

Anke, M., Drobner, C., Röhrig, B., Schäfer, U. and Müller, R. (2002) The selenium content of the flora and plant and animal foodstuffs in Germany. *Ernahrungsforschung,* **47,** 67-79.

Anttolainen, M., Valsta, L.M., Alfthan, G., Keemola, P., Salminen, I. and Tamminen, M. (1996) Effect of extreme fish consumption on dietary and plasma antioxidant levels and fatty acid composition. *Eur. J. Clin. Nutr.* **50**, 741-746.

Aro, A. and Alfthan, G .(1998) Effects of selenium supplementation of fertilisers on human nutrition and selenium status. In: *Environmental Chemistry of Selenium* Eds. WT Frankenberger Jr, RA Engberg, Marcel Dekker, New York. pp81-97.

Aro, A., Alfthan, G. and Varo, P. (1989) Selenium supplementation of fertilizers has increased the selenium intake and serum selenium concentration of Finnish people. In: *Selenium in Biology and Medicine*, Ed. A Wendel, Springer-Verlag, New York. pp242-245.

Aro, A., Alfthan, G. and Varo, P. (1995) Effects of supplementation of fertilizers on human selenium status in Finland. *Analyst*, **120**, 841-843

Arteel, G.A., Briviba, K. and Sies, H. (1999). Protection against peroxynitrite. *FEBS Letters*, **445**, 226-230.

Barclay, M.N.I. and MacPherson, A. (1986) Selenium content of wheat flour used in the UK. *J. Sci. Food Agric.* **37**, 1133-1138.

Barclay, M.N.I., MacPherson, A. and Dixon, J. (1995) Selenium content of a range of UK foods. *J. Fd. Comp. Anal.*, **8**, 307-318.

Barrington, J.W., Lindsay, P., James, D., Smith, S. and Roberts, A. (1996). Selenium deficiency and miscarriage: a possible link? *Brit.J. Obstr. Gynaec.* **103**, 130-132.

Barrington, J.W., Taylor, M., Smith, S. and Bowen-Simpkins, P. (1997). Selenium and recurrent miscarriage. *J. Obstr. Gynaec.* **17**, 199-200.

Bates, C.J., Thane, C.W., Prentice, A. and Delves, H.T. (2002) Selenium status and its correlates in a British national diet and nutrition survey: people aged 65 years and over. *J. Trace Elements in Medicine and Biology.* (Cited by Rayman[2])

Baum M.K., Shor-Posner G., Lai S., Zhang G., Lai H., Fletcher M.A., Sauberlich H. and Page J.B. (1997). High risk of HIV-related mortality is associated with selenium deficiency. *Journal of Acquired Immune Deficiency Syndrome* **15**, 370-374.

Beck M.A., Nelson H.K., Shi Q., Van Dael P., Schiffrin E.J., Blum S., Barclay D. and Levander O.A. (2001) Selenium deficiency increases the pathology of an influenza virus infection. *FASEB Journal* **15**, 1481-1483.

Beck M.A., Shi Q., Morris V.C. and Levander O.A. (1995) Rapid genomic evolution of a non-virulent Coxsackievirus B3 in selenium-deficient mice results in selection of identical virulent isolates. *Nature Medicine* 1, 433-436

Behne, D., Duk, M. and Elger, W.(1986) Selenium content and glutathione peroxidase activity in the testis of the maturing rat. *J. Nutr.* **116**, 1442-1447.

Behne, D., Kyriakopoulos, A., Kalcklosh, M., Weiss-Nowak, C., Pfeifer, H., Gessner, H. and Hamel, C. (1997) Two new selenoproteins found in prostatic glandular epithelium and the spermatid nuclei. *Biomedical and Environmental Science.* **10**, 340-345.

Behne, D., Pfeifer, H., Rothlein, D. and Kyriakopoulos, A. (2000)

Cellular and sub-cellular distribution of selenium and selenoproteins. In: *Trace Elements in Man and Animals*, pp29-33. Eds. AM Roussel, A Favier, RA Anderson. Plenum Press, New York.

Behne, D., Weiler, H., Kyriakopoulos, A. (1996) Effects of selenium deficiency on testicular morphology and function in rats. *J. Reprod. Fertil.* **106,** 291-297.

Blot, W.J., Li, J.Y., Taylor, P.R., Guo, W., Dawsey, S., Wang, G.Q., Yang, C.S., Zhang, S.F., Gail, M., Li, G.Y., Liu, B.Q., Tangrea, J., Sun, Y.H., Liu, F., Fraumeni, F. Jr, Zhang, Y.H. and Li, B. (1993) Nutrition intervention trials in Linxian, China: supplementation with specific vitamin/mineral combinations, cancer incidence and disease-specific mortality in the general population. *J. National Cancer Institute,* **85,** 1483-1490.

Bratakos, M.S., Kanaki, H. Vasiliov-Waite, A. and Ioannou, P. (1990) The nutritional selenium status of healthy Greeks. *Sci. Tot. Envir.* **96,** 161-176.

Brooks, J.D., Metter, E.J., Chan, D.W., Sokol, L.J., Landis, P., Nelson, W.G., Muller, D., Andres, R. and Carter, H.B. (2001) Plasma selenium level before diagnosis and the risk of prostate cancer development. *J. Urol.* **166,** 2034-2038.

Brown, K.M. and Arthur, J.R. (2001) Selenium, selenoproteins and human health, a review. *Public Health Nutrition,* **4,** 593-599.

Bugel, S., Sandstrom, B., Larsen, E.H. and Skibsted, L.H. (2002) Is selenium from animal sources bioavailable? Paper presented to the 11th International Symposium on Trace Elements in Man and Animals, Berkeley, California, USA. June 2-6.

Burk, R.F. and Hill, K.E. (1993) Regulation of selenoproteins. *Annual Review of Nutrition,* **13,** 65-81.

Clark, L.C., Coombs, G.F. Jr, Turnbull, B.W., Slate, E.H., Chalker, D.K., Chow, J., Davis, L.S., Glover, R.A., Graham, G.F., Gross, E.G., Congrad, A., Lesher, J.L. Jr, Kim Park, H., Sanders, B.B. Jr, Smith, C.L. and Taylor, R. (1996) for the National Prevention of Cancer Study Group. Effects of selenium supplementation for cancer prevention in patients with carcinoma of the skin: a randomised control trial. *JAMA,* **276,** 1957-1963. (Published erratum in *JAMA,* **277,** 1520).

Cole, D.J.A. (2000) Selenium, the pig and human diet. In: *Concepts in Pig Science 2000.* Eds. TP Lyons, DJA Cole, Nottingham University Press, Nottingham. pp149-158.

Coombs, G.F. Jr (1989) Selenium In: *Nutrition and Cancer Prevention.* Eds. T Moon, M Micozzi, Marcel Dekker, New York. Pp 389-420.

Coombs, G.F. Jr (2001) Selenium in global food systems. *Brit. J. Nutr.* **85,** 517-547.

Coombs, G.F. Jr. and Gray, W.P. (1998) Chemopreventive agents: selenium. *Pharm. Therapeut.* **79,** 179-192.

Coombs, G.F. Jr. and Lu, J. (2001) Selenium as a cancer preventive agent. In: *Selenium: Its Molecular Biology and Role in Human Health,* pp205-218. Ed. DL Hatfield. Kluwer Academic Publishers, Dordrecht, The Netherlands.

Diaz-Alarcon, J.P., Navarro-Alarcon, M., Lopez-Garcia de la Serrana, H. and Lopez-Martinez, M.C. (1996) Determination of selenium in cereals, legumes and dry fruits from southeastern Spain for calculation of daily dietary intake. *Sci. Tot. Envir.* **184,** 183-189.

Diplock, A.T. (1994) Antioxidants and disease prevention. *Molecular Aspects of Medicine,* **15,** 293-376.

Drobner, C., Rohrig, B., Anke, M. and Thomas, B. (1997) Selenium intake of adults in Germany depending on sex, time, living area and type of diet. In: *Trace Elements in Man and Animals-9: Proceedings of the Ninth International Symposium on Trace Elements in Man and Animals.* Eds. PWF Fischer, MR L'Abbe, KA Cockell, RS Gibson. NRC Research Press, Ottawa, Canada. pp158-159.

Ducros, V., Faure, P., Ferry, M., Couzy, F., Biajoux, I., and Favier, A. (1997) The sizes of the exchangeable pools of selenium in elderly women and their relation to institutionalisation. *Brit. J. Nutr.,* **78,** 379-396.

Duffield-Lillico, A.J., Reid, M.E., Turnbull, B.W., Coombs, G.F. Jr, Slate, E.H., Fischbach, L.A., Marshall, J.R. and Clark, L.C. (2002) Baseline characteristics and the effect of selenium supplementation on cancer incidence in a randomised clinical trial: A summary report of the National Prevention of Cancer Trial. *Cancer Epidemiology Biomarkers and Prevention,* **11,** 630-639.

Dujic, I.S., Dujic, B. and Trajkovic, L. (1995) Dietary intake of selenium in Serbia: results for 1991. *Naucni Skupovi(Srpska AkademijaNauka i Umetnosti) Prirodno MatematickihNauka,* **6,** 81-87.

Edelbauer, A. and Spanischberger, H .(2000) Selenium content in Austrian winter-cereal crops. *Ernahrung,* **24,** 369-376.

El-Bayoumy, K. (1991) The role of selenium in cancer prevention. In: *Practice of Oncology, 4th ed.* Eds. VT Devita, S Hellman, SS Rosenburg, Lippincott, Philadelphia, PA. pp 1-15.

Finley, J.W., Davis, C.D. and Feng, Y. (2000) Selenium from high selenium broccoli protects from colorectal cancer. *J. Nutr.* **130,** 2384-2389.

Ganther, H.E. (1999) Selenium metabolism, selenoproteins and mechanisms of cancer prevention: complexities with thioredoxin reductase. *Carcinogenesis,* **20,** 1657-1666.

Gissel Nielsen, G. (1998) Effects of selenium supplementation of field crops. In: *Environmental Chemistry of Selenium* Eds. WT Frankenberger Jr, RA Engberg, Marcel Dekker, New York. pp99-112.

Gladyshev, V.N. (2001) Identity, evolution and function of selenoproteins and selenoprotein genes. In: *Selenium: Its Molecular Biology and Role in Human Health,* pp99-104. Ed. DL Hatfield. Kluwer Academic Publishers, Dordrecht, The Netherlands.

Gladyshev, V.N., Diamond, A.M. and Hatfield, D.L. (2001) The 15kDa selenoprotein(Sep15): functional studies and a role in cancer etiology. In: *Selenium: Its Molecular Biology and Role in Human Health,* pp99-104. Ed. DL Hatfield. Kluwer Academic Publishers, Dordrecht, The Netherlands.

Golubkina, N.A. (1997) Selenium content in wheat and rye flour from Russia, CSC and Baltic countries. *Voprosy Pitania,* **3, 17-20**.

Golubkina, N.A. (1998) Selenium intake of Briansk region population living in radionuclide-contaminated areas. *Voprosy Pitania,* **4,** 3-6.

Gregory, J., Lowe, S., Bates, C.J., Prentice, A., Jackson, L.V., Smithers, G., Wenlock, R. and Farron, M. (2000) *National Diet and Nutrition Survey: young people aged 4 to 18 years. Volume1.   Report of the diet and nutrition survey.* The Stationery Office, London.

Guimaraes M.J., Peterson D., Vicari V., Cocks B.G., Copeland N.G., Gilbert D.J., Jenkins N.A., Ferrick D.A., Kastelain R.A., Bazan J.F. and Zlotnik A. (1996) Identification of a novel *selD* homolog from Eukaryotes, Bacteria, and Archea: Is there an autoregulatory mechanism in selenocysteine metabolism? *Proceedings of the National Academy of Sciences USA* **93,** 15068-15091

Haldimann, M., Dufosse, K. and Zimmerli, B. (1996) Occurrence of selenium in Swiss cereals. *Mitteilungen aus dem Gebeite der Lebensmitteluntersuchung und Hygiene,* **87,** 267-295.

Hansson, L., Johansson, K., Olin, A. and Siman, G. (1994) Method for the determination of selenium in low-selenium grain and the effect of liming on the uptake of selenium by barley and oats. *Acta Agric. Scand. B. Soil Plant Sci.* **44,** 193-200.

Hartley, W.J. (1963) Selenium and ewe fertility. *Proc. N.Z. Soc. Anim. Prod.* **23**, 20-27.

Health Bulletin; **53,** 294-298.

Hidiroglou, M. (1979) Trace element deficiencies and fertility in ruminants: a review. *J. Dairy Sci.,* **62,** 1195-1206.

Ip, C. (1998) Lessons from basic research in selenium and cancer prevention. *J. Nutr.* **128,** 1845-1854.

Ip, C. and Ganther, H. (1990) Activity of methylated forms of selenium in cancer prevention. *Cancer Research,* **50,** 1206-1211.

Ip, C., Thompson, H.J., Zhu, Z. and Ganther, H.E. (2001) In vitro and in vivo studies of methylselenic acid: evidence that a monomethylated selenium metabolite is critical for cancer chemoprevention. *Cancer Research,* **60,** 2882-2886.

Iwanier K. and Zachara B.A.. (1995) Selenium supplementation enhances the element concentration in blood and seminal fluid but does not change the spermatozoal quality characteristics in subfertile men. J Androl., **16,** 441-447.

Jackson, M.J., Broome, C.S., McArdle, F., Lowe, N.M., Hart, C.A., Kyle, J.A.M. and Arthur, J.R. (2002) Paper presented to the 11th International Symposium on Trace Elements in Man and Animals, Berkeley, California, USA. June 2-6.

Kadrabova, J., Madaric, A. and Ginter, E. (1998) Determination of the daily selenium intake in Slovakia. *Biol. Trace Elem. Res.,* **61,** 277-286.

Kessopoulou, E., Powers, H.J. and Khawam K. (1995) Sharma et al. Treatment of male infertility. *Fertility and Sterility* **64**, No. 4.

Kim, Y.Y. and Mahan, D.C. (2001) Effect of dietary selenium source, level and pig hair colour on various selenium indices. *J. Anim. Sci.,* **79,** 949-955.

Kiremidjian-Schumacher L., Roy M, Wishe H.I., Cohen M.W. and Stotzky G. (1994) Supplementation with selenium and human immune cell functions. *Biological Trace Element Research* **41,** 115-127.

Klapek, T., Mandic, M.L., Grigic, J., Primorac, L., Ikic, M., Lovric, T., Grigic, Z. and Herceg, Z. (1998). Daily dietary intake of selenium in Eastern Croatia. *Science of the Total Environment,* **217,** 127-136.

Knekt, P., Marniemi, J., Teppo, L., Heliovaara, M. and Aromaa, A. (2000) Is low selenium status a risk factor for lung cancer? *Am. J. Epidem.* **148,** 975-982.

Kok, F.J., de Bruijn, A.M., Hofman, A., Vermeeren, R. and Valkenburg, H.A. (1987) Is serum selenium a risk factor for cancer in men only? *Am. J. Epidem.* **125,** 12-16.

Kopicova, Z., Turek, B., Jersukova, V., Vrana, A. and Ksundrova, L. (1992) Selenium content of Foods in the Czech Republic. *Ceskoslovenska Hygiena,* **37,** 101-107.

Korhola, M., Vainio, A. and Edelmann, K. (1986) Selenium yeast. *Annals Clin. Res.,* **18,** 65-68.

Kramer, K., Look, M.P., Chrisafidou, A., Karsten, S. and Areads, J. (1996) Selen und tumarerkrankugen (Selenium and tumorigenesis). *Aktuelle Errnnahrungsmedizin* **21,** 103-113.

Kukreja R and Khan A. (1998) Effect of selenium deficiency and its supplementation on DTH response, antibody forming cells and antibody titre. *Indian Journal of Experimental Biology* **36,** 203-205.

Kumpulainen, J.T., (1993) Selenium in food and diet of selected countries. *J. Trace Elem.Electrol. Health Disease,* **7,** 107-108.

Kvícala, J. and Kroupova, V. (1999). Plasma and urine selenium of cows from various regions of the Czech Republic and its comparison with corresponding human population selenium indexes. In:*Trace Elements in Man and Animals-10*. Eds. AM Roussel, RA Anderson, AE Favier, Kluwer Academic/Plenum Publishing, New York pp.477-478.

Kvícala, J., Zamrazil, V. and Jiránek, V. (2000) Serum and urine selenium changes in a group of elderly during one year of selenium supplementation. In: *Trace Elements in Man and Animals-10*. Eds. AM Roussel, RA Anderson, AE Favier, Kluwer Academic/Plenum Publishing, New York pp417-420.

Lamand, M., Tressol, J.C. and Bellanger, J. (1994) The mineral trace element composition in French food items and intake levels in France. *J. Trace. Elem. Electrol. Health Dis.* **8,** 195-202.

Lyons, T.P., Oldfield, J.E. (1996) The case for organic selenium. *Bull. Selenium-Tellurium Devel. Assoc.,* June, 1-3.

MacPherson, A., Kelly, E.F., Chalmers, J.S., and Roberts, D.J. (1987) The effect of selenium deficiency on fertility in heifers. In: *Trace Substances in Environmental Health – XXI*. Ed.DD Hempill, University of Missouri, Columbia, Missouri, USA. pp551-555.

MAFF (1999). 1997 Total Diet Study – Aluminium, Arsenic, Cadmium, Chromium, Copper, Lead, Mercury, Nickel, Selenium, Tin and Zinc. *Food Surveillance Information Sheet No. 191*. Joint Food Safety and Standards Group, London.

MAFF (1997) Dietary intake of selenium. *Food Surveillance Information Sheet No. 126*. Joint Food Safety and Standards Group, London.

Mahan, D.C., Cline, T.R., and Richert, B. (1999) Effects of dietary levels of selenium-enriched yeast and sodium selenite as selenium sources fed to grower-finishing pigs on performance, tissue selenium, serum glutathione peroxidase activity, carcass characteristics and loin quality. *J. Anim. Sci.,* **77,** 2172-2179.

Mannisto, S., Alfthan, G., Virtanen, M., Kataja, V., Uusitupa, M. and Pietinen, P. (2000) Toenail selenium and breast cancer – a case control study in Finland. *Eur. J. Clin. Nutr.* **54,** 98-103.

Marzec, Z (1999) Analytical and estimated values of chromium, nickel and selenium intakes with adult daily food rations.*BromatologiChemicale Toksykologi,* **32,** 185-189.

McKenzie, R.C., Rafferty, T.S. and Beckett, G.J. (1998) Selenium: an essential element for immune function. *Trends in Immunology Today* **19,** 342-345.

Molnar, J., Drusch, S. and MacPherson, A. (1997) The effect of level and form of supplementary selenium on tissue concentrations in lambs and their importance in raising human dietary selenium intake. In: *Trace Elements in Man and Animals-9: Proceedings of the Ninth International Symposium on Trace Elements in Man and Animals*. Eds. P.W.F. Fischer, M.R. L'Abbe, K.A. Cockell, R.S. Gibson. NRC Research Press,

Ottawa, Canada. pp468-470.

Nicoll, A.E., Norman, J., MacPherson, A. and Acharya, U. (1999). Association of reduced selenium status in the aetiology of recurrent miscarriage. *Brit. J. Obstr. Gynaec.* **106,** 1188-1191.

Noack-Fuller G., De Beer C. and Seibert H. 1993 Cadmium, Lead, selenium, and zinc in semen of occupationally unexposed men. *Andrologia,* **25,** 7-12

Oldereid N.B., Thomassen Y. and Purvis K. (1998) Selenium in human male reproductive organs. Human Reprod. **13,** 2172-2176.

Ortman, K. and Pehrson, B. (1997) Selenite and selenium yeast as feed supplements for dairy cows. *J. Vet. Medic.* **A44,** 373-380.

Parr, R.M., Abdulla, M., Aras, N.K., Byrne, A.R., Camara-Rica, C., Finnie, S., Gharib, A.G., Ingrao, G., Iyengar, G.V., Khangi, F.A., Krishnan, S.S., Kumpulainen, J., Liu, S., Schelenz, R., Srianujata, S., Tanner, J.T. and Wolf, F. (1991) Dietary intakes of trace elements and related nutrients in eleven countries. Preliminary results from an Atomic Energy Agency (IAEA) co-ordinated research programme. In: *Trace Elements in Man and Animals-7* Ed. B Momcilovic, IMI, Zagreb pp13-3-13-5.

Pfeifer, H., Conrad, M., Rothlein, D., Kyriakopoulos, A., Brielmeier, M., BornKamm, G.W.,and Behne, D. (2001) Identification of a specific sperm nuclei selenoenzyme necessary for protamine thiol cross-linking during sperm maturation. *FASEB J.* **15,** 1236-38.

Ratnasinghe, D., Tangrea, J.A., Forman, M.R., Hartman, T., Gunter, E.W., Qiao, Y-L, Yao, S-X, Barett, M.J., Giffen, C.A., Erozan, Y., Tockman, M.S. and Taylor, P.R. (2000) Serum tocopherols, selenium and lung cancer risk among tin miners in China. *Cancer Causes and Control,* **11,** 129-135.

Rayman M.P. (2000). The importance of selenium to human health. Lancet Jul 15; 356(9225): 233-41.

Rayman, M. (2002) The argument for increasing selenium intake. *Review presented to Nutr. Soc.*

Reid, M.E., Duffield-Lillico, A.J., Garland, L., Turnbull, B.W., Clark, L.C. and Marshall, J.R. (2002) Selenium supplementation and lung cancer incidence: an update of the nutritional prevention of cancer trial. *Cancer Epidemiology Biomarkers and Prevention,* **11,** 1285-1291.

Reis, M.F., Holzbecher, J., Martinho, E. and Chatt, A. (1990) Determination of selenium in duplicate diets of residents of Pinhel, Portugal, by neutron activation. *Biol. Trace Elem. Res.* **26,** 629-635.

Robberecht, H.J., Van Cauwenbergh, R. and Deelstra, H.A. (1994) Actual daily dietary intake of selenium in Belgium using duplicate portion sampling. *Zeitschrift fur Lebensmittel*

Untersuchung und Forschung, **199,** 251-254.

Roy, M., Kiremidjian-Schumacher, L., Wishe, H.I., Cohen, M.W. and Strotsky, G. (1994) Supplementation with selenium and human immune cell functions. 1. Effect on lymphocyte proliferation and interleukin 2 receptor expression. *Biol Trace Elem. Res.* **41,** 103-114.

Roy, M., Kiremidjian-Schumacher, L., Wishe, H.I., Cohen, M.W. and Strotsky, G. (1995) *Proc. Soc. Exper. Biol. Med.* **209,** 369-375.

Sanders D.E. (1984) Use of selenium in problem cattle herds. *Modern Veterinary Practice* **65,** 136-138.

Schwartz, K. and Foltz, S.M.. (1957) Selenium as an integral part of factor 3 against necrotic liver degeneration. *J. Mountain Chemical Society,* **79,** 3292-3.

Scott, R., MacPherson, A. and Yates, R.W. (1998). The effect of oral selenium supplementation on human sperm motility. *Br J Urol.,* **82,** 76-80.

Shortt, C.T., Duthie, G.G., Robertson, J.D., Morrice, P.C., Nicol, F. and Arthur, J.R. (1997) Selenium studies of a group of Scottish adults. *Eur. J. Clin. Nutr.* **51,** 1-5.

Sima, A. and Pfannhauser, W. (1998) Selenium levels in foods produced in Austria. In: *Mengen-spurenelem, Arbeitstag 18th*. Ed. M Anke, Verlag Harald Schubert, Leipsig. pp197-204.

Spallholz, J.E., Boylan, L.M. and Larsen, H.S. (1990) Advances in understanding selenium's role in the immune system. *Annals of the New York Academy of Sciences,* **587,** 123-139.

Stadtman, T.C. (1996) Selenocysteine. *Annual Review of Biochemistry,* **65,** 83-100.

Stryer, L. (1995) *Biochemistry,* 4th ed. *p*23. Freeman & Co., New York.

Stuart, L.D. and Oehme, F.W. (1982) Environmental factors in bovine and porcine abortion. *Veterinary and Human Toxicology,* **24,** 435-441.

Sunde, R.A. (1997) Selenium. In: *Handbook of Nutritionally Essential Mineral Elements*, pp493-556. Ed. BL O'Dell and RA Sunde. Marcel Dekker Inc., New York.

Surai, P.F., MacPherson, A., Speake, B.K. and Sparks, N.H.C. (2000) Designer egg evaluation in a controlled trial. *Eur. J Clin. Nutr.* **54,** 298-305.

Taylor, E.W. (1995) Selenium and cellular immunity- evidence that selenoproteins may be encoded in the +1 reading frame overlapping the human CD4, CD8 and HLA-DR genes. *Biol. Trace Elem. Res.* **49,** 85-95.

Taylor, E.W. and Nadimpalli, R.G. (1999) Chemoprotective mechanisms of selenium in cancer and AIDS: evidence for the involvement of novel selenoprotein genes. *InFo Onkologi Supplement* **2,** 7-11.

Templeton A. (1995) Infertility – epidemiology, aetiology and effective management.

Thorn, J., Robertson, J., Buss, D.H. and Bunton, N.G. (1978) Selenium in British Food. *Brit. J. Nutr.* **39,** 391-396.

Turner R.J. and Finch J.M. (1991) Selenium and the immune response. *Proceedings of the Nutrition Society* **50,** 275-285.

Tveitnes, S., Singh, B.R. and Ruud, L. (1996) Selenium concentration in spring wheat as influenced by basal application and top dressing of selenium-enriched fertilizers. *Fertilizer Research,* **45,** 163-167.

Ursini, F., Heim, S., Keiss, M., Maiorino, M., Roveri, A. Wissing, J. and Flohe, L. (1999) Dual function of selenoprotein PHGPx during sperm maturation. *Science,* **285,** 1393-96.

Watanabe, T. and Endo, E. (1991) Effects of selenium deficiency on sperm morphology and spermatocyte chromasomes in mice. *Mutation Res.* **262,** 93-99.

Wilkins, J.F. and Kilgour, R.J. (1982) Production responses to selenium in northern New South Wales. 1. Infertility in ewes and associated production. *Aust. J. Exper. Agric. Anim. Husb.* **22,** 18 –23.

Wingler, K., Bocher, M., Flohe, L., Kollmus, H. and Brigelius-Flohe, R. (1999) mRNA stability and selenocysteine insertion sequence efficiency rank gastrointestinal glutathione peroxidase high in the hierarchy of selenoproteins. *Eur. J. Biochem.* **259,** 149-157.

Wingler, K., Muller, C., Schmehl, K., Florian, S. and Brigelius-Flohe, R. (2000) Gastrointestinal glutathione peroxidase prevents transport of lipid hydroperoxides in CaCo-2 cells. *Gastroenterology,* **119,** 420-430.

Wu, A.S.H., Oldfield, J. E., Shull, L.R. and Cheeke, P.R. (1979) Specific effect of selenium deficiency on rat sperm. *Biol. Reprod.* **20,** 793-798.

Xu B., Chia S.E. and Tsakok M. (1993) Trace elements in blood and seminal plasma and their relationship to sperm quality. *Reprod Toxicol* **7,** 613-618.

Yagodin, B.A., Torshin, S.P., Zabrodina, I . and Yu Dudetskii, A.A. (1999) Accumulation of selenium in spring wheat plants in relation to nutritional conditions. *Agrokhimiya,* **6,** 66-73.

Yoshida, M., Fukinaga, K., Tsuchita, H. and Yasumoto, K. (1999) An evaluation of the bioavailability of selenium in high-selenium yeast. *J. Nutr. Sci. Vitaminol. (Tokyo),* **45,** 119-128.

Yoshizawa, K., Willett, W.C., Morris, S.J., Stampfer, M.J., Spiegleman, D., Rimm, E.B. and Giovanucci, E. (1998) Study of prediagnostic selenium levels in toenails and the risk of advanced prostate cancer. *J. National Cancer Institute,* **90,** 1219-1224.

Yu M-W., Horng I-S., Chiang Y-C., Liaw Y-F. and Chen C-J. (1999)

Plasma selenium levels and the risk of hepatocellular carcinoma among men with chronic hepatitis virus infection. *American Journal of Epidemiology* **150,** 367-74.

Yu S.Y., Zhu Y.J. and Li W.G. (1997) Protective role of selenium against hepatitis B virus and primary liver cancer in Quidong. *Biological Trace Element Research* **56,** 117-124.

Benefits and sources of antioxidation in pet food

Lucy Tucker and Hans-Peter Healy

Companion animal nutrition has seen advances in the understanding and application of the correct balance of nutrients required in the diet during the last decade. Consumers expect pet food, even budget ranges, to consistently high quality. Oxidation causes rancidity, making pet food unappetising and reducing nutritional value. It also increases the levels of oxidising materials (referred to as 'free radicals' or 'reactive oxygen species'), which cause various metabolic and physiological diseases. For these reasons, and because pet food utilises high fat raw materials, such as animal meals, animal fats and vegetable oils, that are prone to rancidity, stabilisation with suitable and effective antioxidants is important. Hence, antioxidation in pet food is concerned with three distinct areas:

- Food stabilisation and quality control
- Maintaining health and longevity in companion animals
- Palatability and sensory attributes

Antioxidant compounds may be of synthetic or natural origin. Due to the ubiquitous problems of oxidation, from necessary processes in the body and external sources such as UV light, plants and animals have developed strategies to reduce these harmful effects. Naturally occurring antioxidants from plant materials are available as commercial products developed for use in pet foods. Manufacturers should consider the forms of antioxidants available, in order to ensure high quality, long shelf life of dry pet food and also take advantage of marketing opportunities afforded by the use of more natural ingredients.

The importance of anti-oxidation in pet food manufacture

It is not feasible to make a commercial dry or baked pet food without incorporating antioxidants. Pet foods are particularly dependent on these compounds, especially considering the typical requirement for twelve to eighteen months shelf life. Factors contributing to fat rancidity, and the outcomes of this damage are given below (Figure 1).

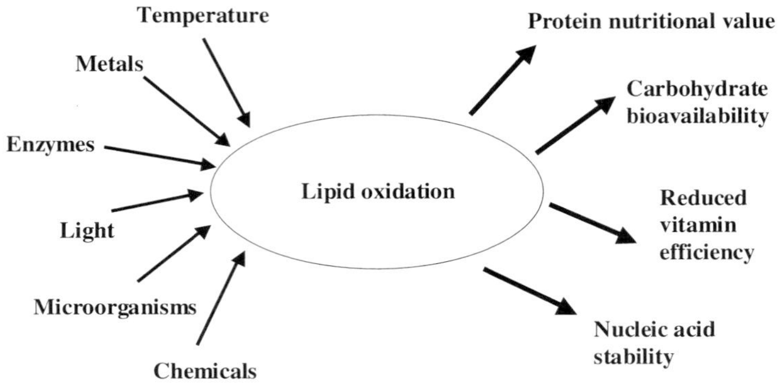

Figure 1.
Causes and effects of oxidative rancidity

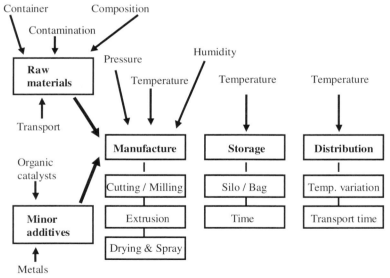

Considerable stresses are induced during the manufacturing processes in all market categories of pet foods, whether stabilized naturally or synthetically. (Figure 2) summarises where these stresses occur during pet food processing.

Figure 2.
Initiation of oxidative rancidity in food manufacturing

Antioxidant compounds protect pet food formulations from the deleterious effects of autoxidation that begins when lipid radicals are produced by hydrolytic oxidation of fatty acids. These combine with oxygen to form free radicals that ultimately break down fats, causing rancid odours, reduced shelf life, poor palatability and texture, reduced nutritional value, low quality and potentially, toxicity. Antioxidants react with free radicals, negating their potency and so preserve pet food quality.

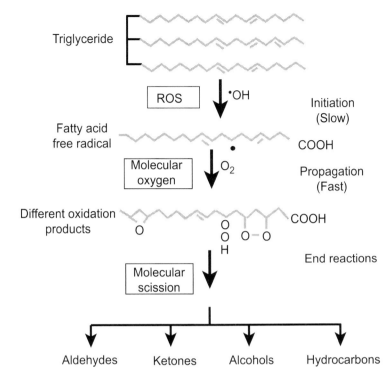

Figure 3.
Molecular steps
of oxidative
rancidity

Preventing rancidity in foods can be achieved by applying certain conditions during manufacturing (Table 1), however the only viable alternative is the application of antioxidants.

Table 1.
Strategies to
reduce
oxidation in
food
manufacture
(adapted from
Laue, 2006)

Strategy	Suitability for pet food manufacture
Low temperature	Not possible due to legislation
	Clean-room process potentially expensive
Oxygen subtraction	Difficult to implement, more expensive process
	Requires specific packaging
Metal chelation	More expensive ingredients
Antioxidation	Highly efficient, easily incorporated, relatively inexpensive

Successfully stabilizing pet food is a complicated exercise, beginning with the selection and management of raw materials. Because of the nature of some of the raw materials typically used from the rendering industry, variability in product quality and stability can be difficult. The rendering industry uses materials from slaughter plants, which are high in minerals (blood, bones, etc.) that are associated with free radical generation. Stabilizing these materials takes research, expertise and constant monitoring. Additionally, the physical nature of many meat meals as dried powders offers large surface areas with high exposure to oxygen, increasing the potential for oxidation.

Premium pet food contains higher levels of polyunsaturated vegetable oils and fats, which are more difficult to stabilise, and increase the overall demand for antioxidants. Processing methods, such as grinding, pre-conditioning, extruding, coating, drying and cooling, all increase exposure of raw materials to heat or oxygen, initiating oxidation. Understanding how these reactions impact the raw materials and antioxidant system is crucial in designing a successful custom antioxidant program for each formulation.

Antioxidation in companion animals

Oxidation is a necessary phenomenon of cell functions, as oxygen is utilised in respiration, metabolism and energy production. Oxygen is highly reactive and potentially toxic (Knight, 1998), and fundamental biochemical mechanisms, such as respiration, result in the production of oxidizing compounds, the majority being in the chemical form O_2^-. These are highly unstable, and facilitate various chain reactions, which can damage cell membranes and tissue function. Free radicals have been identified as causative agents for pulmonary hypertension syndrome (ascites), inflammation, arteriosclerosis, neoplastic diseases, cataracts, cancerous tumour development and various reproductive disorders. Free radicals reduce cell function and interfere with growth by damaging DNA, proteins, lipids (and hence membranes) and carbohydrates, which is why they are linked to such a wide variety of ailments and disorders.

Companion animals show more variability in their levels of oxidative stress than farm animals, primarily due to the wide range of uses and demands placed upon them. Adequate antioxidant supply is still very important regardless of the source of oxidative stress, as the effect is the same. Long-lived animals have an increased requirement for a ready supply of effective antioxidants to ensure disease resistance, cellular repair and non-clinical tissue maintenance. Cancer is a major killer of dogs and cats, primarily due to their long lives and exposure to oxidative stress. DNA damaged by oxidising materials can fail to replicate correctly, leading to tumour growth. Increases in oxidative stress can come from varying quarters, and, in pet species, are often a result of their urban or household environment (Table 2).

Internally oxidising stresses	External oxidising sources
Respiration – mitochondria	Cigarette smoke
Immunity - phagocytes	Radiation
Reactions with transition	UV light
metals (e.g. Fe)	Pollution
Pro-oxidant inorganic elements	Certain drugs
Arachidonate pathways	Chemical reagents
Peroxisomes	Industrial solvents
Under/over exercising	Mycotoxins in cereals
Inflammation	Oxidised dietary fat
Vaccination	Disease challenges

Antioxidants can be associated with anti-inflammatory activity. A good example of this is the phytogenic compound, silymarin, which has been widely demonstrated to reduce arthritic and oedemal inflammation in both humans and rodents (Skidmore-Roth, 2001).

Under normal, unstressed physiological conditions, it has been estimated that between 3 and 5% of cellular oxygen is transformed into free radicals (Singal et al, 1998), an amount which increases dramatically during stress (e.g. disease, hard physical work). If the immune system is stimulated, free radicals are produced in large amounts during the proliferation of immune cells, and are used to damage and inactivate invading pathogens (Schwartz, 1996; Kettle & Winterburn, 1997), but will also cause damage to internal structures in the animal unless they are removed efficiently.

Organisms have evolved specific antioxidant protective mechanisms that helped them to survive in the atmosphere when oxygen concentration was rising (Halliwell and Gutteridge, 1999). As a result there are thousands of naturally occurring compounds possessing antioxidant properties to disable free radicals. These compounds work in various ways – as shown in table 3, however the main modes of action can be split into three.

1. Prevention of initial free radical formation. This is achieved by binding to co-factors required for formation of free radicals, such as iron. However, as we have seen from the immune example above, most reactions that generate free radicals are very important, so this is not always desirable.

2. Binding excess free radicals once they have been formed. This can be seen with nutrients such as vitamins C and E, and prevent the initiation of cascade reactions.

3. Antioxidant enzyme system in cells. These enzymes work as a team with the chelating antioxidants by 'recycling' them – i.e.

removing and neutralising the bound radicals to allow the chelating agents to function fully again. They can also include the 'repair' enzymes that reverse damage caused by free radicals.

Two main enzymes are involved in effective antioxidation; superoxide dismutase (SOD) and glutathione peroxidase (GSH-Px). Certain minerals are integral components of these enzymes and are required in sufficient amounts from the diet to ensure synthesis in cell organelles to maximise the efficiency of anti-oxidation, for example GSH-Px is highly dependant on selenium for its synthesis. There are two major forms of SOD in the cell: manganese-SOD (located in mitochondria) and copper or zinc-SOD (found in the cytosol). This enzyme transforms the O_2^- free radical to form hydrogen peroxide (H_2O_2), rather than the more reactive radicals such as hydroxyl free radical OH*, which would occur otherwise.

$$O_2^- + O_2^- + 2H^+ \xrightarrow{\text{SOD}} H_2O_2 + O_2$$

H_2O_2 is more stable, but still toxic and must be removed from the cell by a further reaction shown below, facilitated by either GSH-Px or catalase (CAT). Because GSH-Px is found in many cellular locations while CAT is located mainly in peroxisomes, the efficacy of H_2O_2 removal from the cell is greater with GSH-Px.

$$H_2O_2 \xrightarrow{\text{GSH-Px}} H_2O$$

This first level of antioxidant defence in the cell is not sufficient to completely prevent free radical formation and lipid peroxidation, therefore a second level of antioxidant defence includes fat-soluble (vitamins A, E, carotenoids, ubiquinols) and water-soluble (e.g. ascorbic acid, glutathione, uric acid) antioxidants. These antioxidants are potent chain-breaking compounds, which prevent free radical propagation. This mechanism is not straightforward, for example vitamin E reacts with a lipid peroxyl radical (LOO*), becomes oxidised, and lipid hydroperoxide (LOOH) is produced in the following reaction:

$$\text{Vitamin E} + \text{LOO*} \longrightarrow \text{Vitamin E-radical} + \text{LOOH}$$

Lipid hydroperoxide products can react with metals such as iron to form cytotoxic products such as aldehydes, alkoxyl radicals (LO*) and peroxyl radicals (LOO*):

$$LOOH + Fe^{2+} \longrightarrow LO^* + Fe^{3+} + OH^-$$
$$LOOH + Fe^{3+} \longrightarrow LOO^* + Fe^{2+} + H^+$$

Table 3. Common antioxidant compounds and pre-cursors

Antioxidant	Action	Source	Availability	Problems
Vitamin E	Chain breaking antioxidant	Plant oils, fat soluble	Liver & adipose body reserves	Unstable, expensive, stable ester needs metabolic conversion
Vitamin C	Vitamin E recycling	Citrus fruit, plants	Synthesis *in vivo*	Unstable, poor storage, high excretion rate
Carotenoids	Immune system modulation	Plant pigments	Dietary supplement, maize	Unstable, limited body storage
Glutathione	Cellular enzymes GSH-Px	Synthesis *in vivo*	Cell organelles	Ineffective as dietary supplement
Selenium	Key component GSH-Px. Trace element	Plant (esp. cereal) intake EU deficiency	Organic Se-yeast stored in body Inorganic Na - selenite	Selenite – pro-oxidant. Toxic at high dose. Poor absorption.
Zinc	Cellular enzymes – SOD Trace element		Inorganic – poor storage.	Inorganic Zn – poor efficacy
Copper	Cellular enzymes – SOD	Dietary minerals & supplementation	Organic forms – good uptake & tissue	Inorganic form – pro-oxidant
Manganese	Cellular enzymes - SOD			Inorganic form – poor uptake
Iron	Cellular enzymes – Catalase			Inorganic form – strong pro-oxidant. Vitamin & lipid damage – must be bound to protein

Again, GSH-Px is required to negate lipid hydroperoxides. This second level of antioxidant defence is not entirely able to prevent lipid peroxidation, and some biological molecules will become damaged. In this case the third level of antioxidant defence deals with the repair of damaged molecules, consisting of specific enzymes such as proteases or lipases.

This interaction between the different antioxidant systems demonstrates the importance of 'teamwork' within the body. Whilst each level of anti-oxidation is important in its own right, it is only by ensuring they all work in harmony that complete protection can be afforded to the animal. It also ensures the efficient use of antioxidant resources that are often poorly stored in the body or in limited supply, such as the recycling of vitamin E.

The requirement a pet has for antioxidants varies from one individual to another and is dependant upon the age, breed, health, work rate, physiological status, welfare and environment that pet is kept in. Exposure to city pollution, or in the case of some pets cigarette smoke, are all generators of oxidative stress. This makes it essential to supply adequate levels of antioxidant and precursor components for SOD, GSH-Px and CAT in a dietary form that is readily absorbed and stored in the body. When the oxidative stress level changes, the body is then prepared to deal with free radicals effectively before any serious damage occurs.

Fat-soluble antioxidants, such as vitamin E and carotenoids, operate within lipid-rich membranes and tissues primarily, whereas water-soluble ascorbic acid (vitamin C) and glutathione can be synthesised in the body and require adequate supply of basic components via the diet. Transition elements are necessary for synthesis of key antioxidant enzymes; Se is essential for GSH-Px. Zinc, copper and manganese form integral parts of SOD and iron is a component of catalase. Deficiency (and in some cases excess) of these elements causes oxidative stress and damage to biological structures. Selenium deficiency is a particular problem, as the main dietary sources are plants that must grow in selenium-rich soils to accumulate the element. European soils are very low in selenium, and intakes in both the human and animal population have been declining in recent decades.

The use of inorganic sources of elements such as zinc has been found to be less well absorbed, stored and utilised compared to organic forms (amino acid chelates) of these metals. This is because animals have evolved mechanisms to extract organic forms from their diet, usually bound to amino acids (Surai, 2000). An example of this is the organic selenium synthesised and stored in certain yeasts, which is in the form of seleno-methionine (as found in plant materials).

Antioxidant sources

Antioxidants can be divided into two distinct categories: synthetic and natural. Synthetic compounds have been commercially available to manufacturers for many years and form an inexpensive, reliable way of stabilising pet foods. More recently, certain sectors of consumers have increased the demand for 'natural foods', which do not contain chemical compounds, but rather utilise naturally occurring ingredients. Within this consumer group, the interest in using antioxidants derived from plant materials has increased, and is used as a marketing tool.

Antioxidants are present within raw materials used in the diet, and can provide a useful level of protection (Figure 4). However these are insufficient to stabilise the complete diet.

Figure 4. Levels of naturally occurring vitamin E in vegetable raw materials (Laue, 2006)

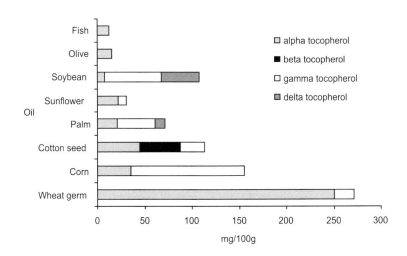

Synthetic antioxidants

Synthetic antioxidant compounds have a phenolic structure and include butylated hydroxyanisole (BHA), butylated hydroxytoluene (BHT) and ethoxyquins. Figure 5 shows how they bind and negate the effects of free radicals in food.

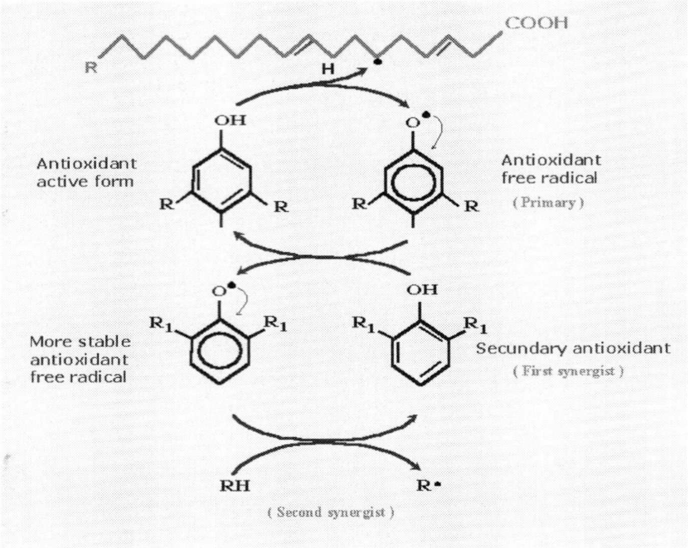

Figure 5.
Mechanism
of action of a
synthetic
antioxidant

Reports (Dzanis, 1991) regarding the safety of using ethoxyquin led the FDA in 1997 to request the pet food industry to voluntarily reduce its inclusion from a level of 150 ppm to 75 ppm, limiting its usefulness. Factors such as this, combined with an increasing trend among informed consumers seeking natural foods, have led to a swing from synthetic antioxidant usage in the industry. BHA and BHT continue to be regarded as highly effective antioxidants, and are commonly used in commercial pet food.

Natural antioxidants

There is a selection of natural antioxidant products commercially available for use in pet foods. Certain phytogenic ingredients show strong antioxidant properties, and form the focus of research (especially regarding human health) as potential food and feed supplements. Hops, rosemary, thyme, turmeric and grapeseed extracts show interesting levels of anti-oxidation activity via free radical chelation in vitro, whereas other plant-derived antioxidants operate through repair or chain-breaking mechanisms (Table 4).

The chemical form of the antioxidant dictates its mode of action. Figures 6 and 7 below show the various forms of extracts from rosemary, which chelate free radicals in a similar manner to synthetic phenolic compounds.

152

Plant	Active ingredient	Mode of action
Milk thistle	Silymarin	RNA polymerase repair, Anti-peroxide & aldehyde
Hops	Humelone, Buteneol	Chelator, heat stable
Lemon Balm	Polyphenols	Chelator
Tomato/ Water melon	Lycopene	Chain breaking
Grapeseed Cranberry Rosemary	Phenols	Chelator
Paprika	Capisxanthin	Immune system, chelator
Marigold	Lutein	Immune system, chelator
Thyme	Glutatione peroxidase	Anti-oxidant precursor

Table 4. Phytogenic sources of antioxidants

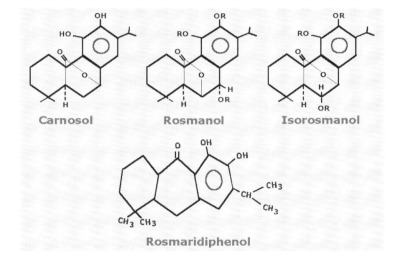

Figure 6. Structure of antioxidant compounds found in the plant rosemary (Laue, 2006)

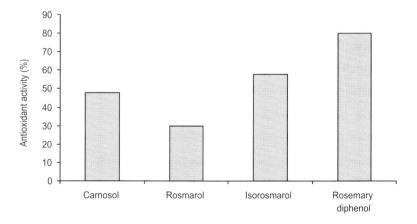

Figure 7. Antioxidant activity of extracts from rosemary (Laue, 2006)

The pet food industry started supplementing with natural antioxidants in the mid-1990's, and their use has expanded rapidly. Today, premium pet food predominantly contains mixed tocopherols (vitamin E) and rosemary extracts (singly or in combination) to stabilize individual raw materials such as animal fats, vegetable and fish oils, meats, meat meals and fish and complete pet foods. Chelating agents, such as citric acid (vitamin C), can be used to bind free metals, especially iron and copper, which promote oxidation. Ideally, non-charged forms of organic minerals (such as proteinated chelates) should be included in the feed to reduce the negative impact of inorganic trace elements.

Maintaining pet food stability through antioxidants

A major issue for antioxidants in pet food manufacturing is their stability during processing. Certainly, the instability of vitamin C has been well documented, and alternatives may be used to boost total antioxidant levels in pet food. Some of the phytogenic materials, such as hops, show good, even improved, stability on heating.

Case studies examining antioxidant requirements for pet food samples with confirmed rancidity, have shown how certain raw materials can contribute to increase oxidation. Pet food E (Figure 8) was found to be consistently rancid, and a five-day Schaal oven test revealed that pet foods A, E and F were unstable, as seen in the high peroxide values (PV) for these samples.

Figure 8.
Peroxide values
for six
commercial pet
foods

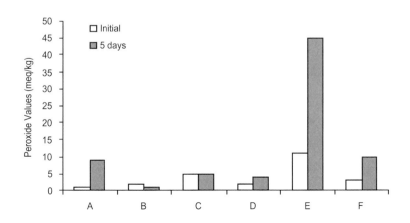

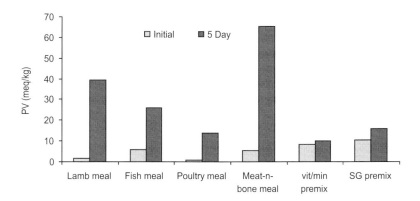

Figure 9.
Initial and five
day peroxide
value test results
in incoming raw
materials

Testing individual raw materials for PV after 5 days revealed that
the lamb meal, fish meal and meat & bone meal were the most
likely sources of oxidation (Figure 9). In addition, the flaxseed oil
(Figure 10) was found to contain no antioxidants and was unstable
on delivery. Some materials had only been treated with antioxidants
immediately prior to shipping, with the meat and bone meal being
approximately two to four days old at this stage. New protocols
were established for the rendering company, which eliminated
oxidative damage. Similar arrangements were made with the fish
meal, lamb meal and flaxseed oil suppliers. Implementing a new
custom antioxidant program meant that the stability of the all the
formulations improved dramatically.

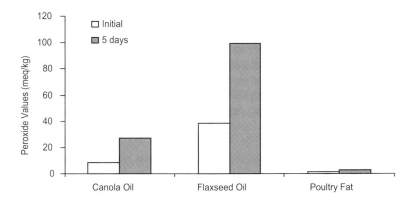

Figure 10.
Peroxide values
for three types of
fat used in pet
food manufacture

Synthetic versus natural antioxidants

There is discussion within the industry regarding the efficacy of
natural antioxidants versus established synthetic versions.
Commercial products are now available that contain a blend of
natural antioxidants developed specifically for inclusion into pet

food. One such product is Nature Ban™ (Alltech Inc, USA), which contains tocopherols (vitamin E complexes), rosemary extracts and citric acid (vitamin C). This combination shows increased and potentially synergistic antioxidant activity, compared to the activity of its constituent compounds (Figure 11).

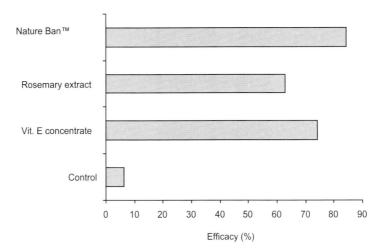

Figure 11. Efficacy of single and combined antioxidant compounds

Trials conducted to examine the efficacy of a natural antioxidant product have shown improved stability of high fat raw materials that often contribute to the problems of rancidity in pet food.

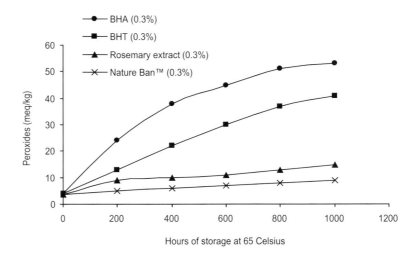

Figure 12a. Stabilisation of soybean meal using different antioxidant products, method AOM, air flow 180 L/h (Valenzuela, 2002)

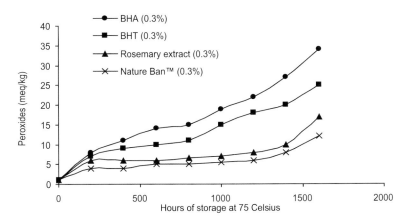

Figure 12b.
Stabilisation of chicken fat meal using different antioxidant products, method AOM, air flow 180 L/h (Valenzuela, 2002)

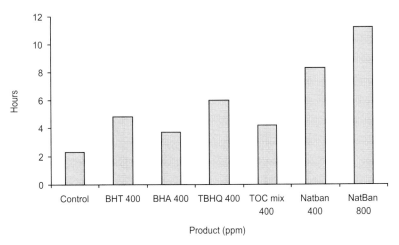

Figure 12c.
Stability characteristics of fish oils (by Rancimet analysis) using different antioxidant products (Valenzuela, 2002)

Stability and application

Heat tolerance is a key attribute for natural alternatives to synthetic antioxidants. Research at the University of Santiago in Chile (Valenzuela, 2003) demonstrated that a Nature Ban™ was thermally stable for 1 hour at 200°C and for 2 hours at 150°C when tested on refined sardine oil.

Commercial experience indicates that natural antioxidants are quite heat stable, with losses of less than 30% reported after extrusion. The period of heating caused by extrusion lasts for only a few seconds, however, this loss needs to be taken into consideration and compensated for when formulating an antioxidant program. Losses of less than 20% have been seen in baked dog foods, which undergo extensive periods of heating. The cooling of pet foods to ambient air temperatures before bagging is important, but in practice is frequently not achieved. Kibbles, which are bagged while hot, can stay hot for days especially in the middle of a pallet or bag, which exposes the pet food to further excessive heating. Such issues radically increase oxidative damage and potentially limit the efficacy of heat labile antioxidants such as vitamin C and E.

Many factors must be taken into consideration when designing an antioxidant program for pet food to achieve the desired shelf life and quality. A target level of antioxidant for the finished pet food should be determined, based on the total dietary fat percentage and including compensation for losses due to extrusion. Polyunsaturated fatty acids (e.g. fish oils, canola, flaxseed oils) are more difficult to stabilise, have a higher rancidity potential and so require increased antioxidant levels. High fat diets need different amounts of antioxidants, relative to very low fat diets. If practicable, levels of natural antioxidants present in the raw materials can be taken into consideration, and the supplemented antioxidant product required reduced accordingly.

At the pet food plant level, natural antioxidants can be added at numerous points in production, as illustrated by Figure 13. In order to ensure there are sufficient antioxidants to quench free radicals during the extrusion process, additional dry antioxidant supplementation is recommended (via the mineral premix). Meat slurries made from frozen blocks should have liquid natural antioxidant added to protect the meat through processing and extrusion.

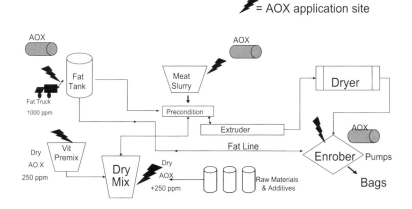

Figure 13. Application points for addition of natural antioxidant products in commercial pet food manufacturing

Conclusions

Antioxidants are required to secure the quality and shelf life of pet food as well as maintaining the health of the animal that receives the food. It is vital that the balance of antioxidant supply in the diet versus oxidising free radical production (both internally and externally generated) must be maintained to ensure protection against cellular degradation and disease. There is no doubt, from the body of research available, that there are many antioxidant feed ingredients with useful and relevant benefits that can be used in pet food. It is crucial to understand which of these alternatives are most suitable to use, via their mode of action and efficacy. Understanding the importance of maintaining sufficient and available levels of antioxidants for companion animals is improving. Correct dietary supplementation with suitable antioxidant sources to prevent oxidative damage in pets is key to maintaining well-being and longevity.

References

Dzanis, D.A. (1991). Safety of Ethoxyquin in dog foods. *J. Nutr*, **21**: S163

Furst, P. (1996). The role of antioxidants in nutritional support. *Proceedings of the Nutrition Society* **55** (3): 945-961

Halliwell, B. & Gutteridge, J.M.C. (1999). *Free Radicals in Biology and Medicine* Third Edn, Oxford University Press, Oxford

Kettle, A.J. & Winterburn, C.C. (1997). Mierloperoxidase: a key regulator of neutrophil oxidant production. *Redox Report*, **3**: 3-15

Knight, J.A. (1998). Free radicals: their history and current status in aging and disease. *Annals of Clinical and Laboratory Science* **28** (6): 331-346

Laue, D-K. (2006). Personal communication

Schwartz, K.B. (1996). Oxidative stress during viral infection: a review. *Free Radical Biology and Medicine* **21**: 641-649

Singal, P.K., Khaper, N., Palace, V. and Kumar, D. (1998). The role of oxidative stress in the genesis of heart disease *Cardiovascular Research* **43** (1): 248-249

Skidmore-Roth, L. (2001) *Handbook of Herbs and Natural Supplements* Mosby Inc, St Louis, USA

Surai P.F. (2000). Organic selenium: benefits to animals and humans, a biochemist's view. In: *Biotechnology In The Feed Industry*. Proc. Of The 16th Annual Symposium (T.P.Lyons And K.A. Jacques, Eds.). Nottingham University Press, Nottingham, UK, Pp.205-260..

Valenzuela, A. (2002). Natural antioxidants: from food safety to health benefits. *Proceedings of the 18ᵗʰ Alltech International Symposium* Kentucky, USA P 323-332

Valenzuela, A., Nieta, S., Sanhueza, J. & Gomez-Basauri, J. (2003). Chemical and physical properties of a new food-grade antioxidant: Preventox™ *Proceedings of the 19ᵗʰ Alltech International Symposium* Kentucky, USA pp. 379-384

Water activity as a tool for predicting and controlling the stability of pet foods

R.A. Timmons

Introduction: water activity defined

'Food safety' was one of many buzz phrases for 2005. As 2006 rolls forward, we can see that the attention focused on the safety of food is here to stay. The Federal Food, Drug, and Cosmetic Act requires that pet foods, like human foods, be pure and wholesome, containing no harmful or deleterious substances. Consumers are becoming increasingly aware of the quality aspects of what they eat, as well as the quality of what they feed their beloved pets. One important aspect of food quality is the stability of the final product. Changes in physical, chemical or microbiological properties of food can be considered loss of stability. Water activity (Aw) is one of several important parameters that affect stability of foods.

Water activity is a measure of the free moisture in a foodstuff. It is also defined as the quotient of the water vapor pressure of the substance divided by the vapor pressure of pure water at the same temperature (US FDA, 2005). Free moisture can be explained as water that is available to participate in physical, chemical and biological reactions. Water activity is not to be confused with moisture content. Moisture content is the combination of free and bound moisture. The relationship between moisture and water activity depends on the specific material. Silicon dioxide, for example, could absorb 50% moisture and maintain a very low water activity while crystalline sucrose absorbs little water until it reaches an Aw of 0.80. Characteristics of individual ingredients can be very important and will be discussed in this paper.

Role of water activity

Microbiological control

Water activity plays a role in the microbial stability of ingredients and final pet foods. Bacteria, molds and yeast require water for growth; and every microorganism has a minimum water activity below which it will not grow. Table 1 details the level of water activity needed to inhibit different types of microorganisms (Fontana, 2000). A water activity of less than 0.85 is needed in food in order to avoid regulatory attention. At a water activity of less than 0.85, a food is considered non-hazardous because there is not enough available water to support pathogen growth.

Table 1.
Microorganisms and the water activities at which they are typically inhibited

Water activity	Microorganisms generally inhibited
0.950	Pseudomonas, Escherichia, Proteus, Bacillus, Clostridium perfringens, some yeasts
0.910	Salmonella, C. botulinum, Lactobacillus, Pediococcus, some molds
0.870	Many yeasts
0.800	Most molds (mycotoxigenic penicillia), Straphylococcus aureus, most Saccharomyces
0.750	Most halophilic bacteria, mycotoxigenic aspergilli
0.650	Xerophilic molds
0.600	Osmophilic yeasts, few molds

Fontana, 2000

Water activities of many common ingredients and categories of pet foods are shown in Table 2. Dry pet food and hard treats typically are in the 0.40-0.45 Aw range. At this low level of available water (< 0.60 Aw), microbial stability is not an issue. Canned foods, however, are typically higher than 0.85 Aw and must be treated as acidified foods. Water activities of less than 0.85, while considered non-hazardous from the standpoint of pathogenic bacterial growth, will still support the growth of many yeasts and molds. Growth of these microorganisms can cause spoilage and physical deterioration. Soft pet foods and kibbles typically fall in this intermediate range (0.60-0.85 Aw). Supplementary processing such as pasteurization, pH control or addition of preservatives is necessary for protection of these foods. It often becomes a formulation tradeoff between maintaining a moist, chewy food and the added costs of preservatives and/or processing.

Table 2.
Water activities of some common foods and ingredients

	Water activity
Canned pet food	0.85 and greater
Soft moist pet food, ~ 22% moisture	0.83
Starch	0.65-0.80
Maple syrup	0.80
Dried whole egg, 10% moisture	0.70
Rolled oats, 10% moisture	0.65
Raw cane sugar	0.65
Dry pet foods	0.40-0.45
Whole egg powder, 5% moisture	0.40

Mold and toxins

Mold can grow at water activity levels as low as 0.61. Types of mold, temperature and water activity play a role in determining growth characteristics. For example, Penicillium roqueforti germinated at 0.82 Aw at 25°C, 0.86 Aw at 30°C and was unable to germinate at 37°C. Eurotium repens germinated at 0.70 Aw at 30°C, but at 25 and 37°C, the minimum water activity for germination was 0.74. These fungi all grew faster under acidic rather than neutral pH conditions (Gock et al., 2003).

Toxins, notably mycotoxins in the case of feedstuffs, may be formed during the course of microbial growth, but not below 0.80 Aw (Lowe and Kershaw, 1995). Formation of mycotoxins depends on the type of mold, substrate and storage conditions, which include pH, temperature and water activity. A test of dry cereal-based pet foods and wild bird seed by Scudamore et al. (1997) for the presence of aflatoxin and ochratoxin found that 84% of these foods contained amounts that were below detectable limits. Ochratoxins were found in 10% of the samples at low levels. Penicillium, Eurotium and Aspergillus were the main genera of mold present on higher moisture samples of the food.

Mycotoxins can be formed on cereal grains such as corn and wheat. Processing temperatures can kill the mold but will not remove toxins that are already formed. Testing of raw materials can help to limit the amount of toxins in food. Sampling can be very difficult because pockets of mold growth, and therefore mycotoxin formation, can occur during storage and transport. Mycotoxin formation can also occur during storage of the final food. Development of mycotoxins can be avoided by keeping the final water activity below 0.8.

Infestation

Insects are another potential problem during storage of pet foods, which in some cases can be controlled by water activity. Mites are commonly found in some food ingredients and have the ability to survive through some processing steps. Mites may be active at 5°C above 0.65 Aw, at 25° above 0.63 Aw and at 40°C above 0.60 Aw (Decagon, 2003). Dry pet foods and treats, which are well below 0.60 Aw, should remain free of mites.

Chemical stability

Water activity also influences chemical stability. Non-enzymatic browning, known as the Maillard reaction, is a chemical reaction between simple sugars and amino acids, which results in increasing color. As Figure 1 illustrates, non-enzymatic browning occurs between Aw 0.3 and 0.8. Browning leads to changes in appearance as well as to the formation of off-flavors. Enzymes can also lead to reactions in food, leading to off-flavors. Enzyme reactions are substantially slowed at water activity levels of 0.8 or lower.

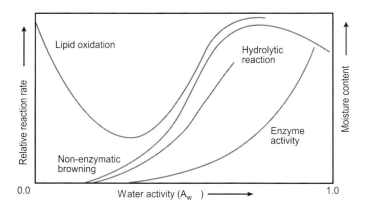

Figure 1.
Reaction rates in foods as a function of water activity

Physical stability

Physical stability is extremely dependent on water activity. Dried foods will come to a final equilibrium with their environment. If the relative humidity of the environment is higher than the equilibrium water activity of the product, the product will take on water until it reaches equilibrium with the environment. If this new water activity is above the critical limit for the food, it will begin to cake, which is unacceptable to the consumer.

A critical water activity limit should be determined for each new product. This can be established by creating a water absorption isotherm (Figure 2). An isotherm is created at a set temperature by examining water activity readings vs. moisture readings for a product. From the isotherm, the water moisture level that the product will reach at a specific relative humidity at a set temperature can be established. If the moisture level associated with the critical limit (physical characteristics change) for a product is noted, storage/packaging conditions can be established. A product with a critical limit above realistic storage conditions will not need special packaging. Products with a lower critical limit might need airtight sealed containers.

Individual ingredients can also affect the final product stability. Ingredients with different initial water activities will come to equilibrium in the product. A spray-dried product with an initial 0.2 Aw mixed with an intermediate ingredient of 0.5 Aw will reach

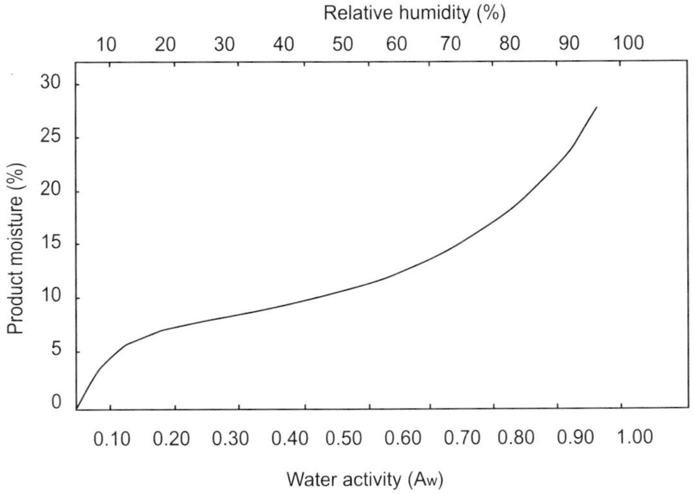

Figure 2.
Typical water
isotherm of a
product.

equilibrium at a value between the two. The higher activity ingredient will lose available water to the lower activity ingredient. The characteristics of each ingredient could change. Again, this depends on the critical limits of each individual ingredient, as well as the critical limit of the final product. Salwin (1963) developed an equation using water activity and moisture from individual component isotherms to predict the water activity of the mixture at equilibrium (Figure 3). In order for the prediction to represent the actual situation, isotherms must be developed at the temperature at which the final product will be held. Packaging should be such that the environmental humidity need not be considered a factor.

Figure 3.
Salwin
equation for
predicting
water activity at
equilibrium

$$A_w = \frac{(W_1 \cdot S_1 \cdot A_{w1}) + (W_2 \cdot S_2 \cdot A_{w2})}{(W_1 \cdot S_1) + (W_2 \cdot S_2)}$$

W_1 = grams solids Ingredient 1
S_1 = linear slope Ingredient 1
A_{w1} = Initial A_w Ingredient 1

It is typical for some pet foods/treats to have a mixture of soft chewy pieces and some harder pieces. The harder pieces are considered valuable for their ability to keep teeth cleaned, while the softer pieces are considered more palatable. When mixed, the two materials will come to equilibrium. In order for this mix to remain stable, the individual components and final product must be developed in order that the final equilibrium water activity will allow the two components to retain their original characteristics. This has been the subject of many patents on both the pet food and human food sides. Specialty packaging, processing and ingredients have all been used in order to obtain the goal of maintaining a stable final product.

Transfer of water between ingredients is a common cause of caking. The transfer of water from an ingredient with higher water activity to an ingredient with a lower water activity causes one of the ingredients to reach its critical limit, initiating caking. Storage factors such as temperature can change the rate of this reaction. Lower temperatures will slow the reaction, while higher temperatures speed reaction rate.

Product development

Food technologists will utilize all of the information above when developing a new product. The first goal is to establish the type of product (low, intermediate, or high moisture) to be produced. Producers of a low moisture food will not need to worry about microbiological issues. Water activity will be a factor in this food with regard to physical characteristics. The Salwin equation in Figure 3 is useful in predicting the final water activity of a mixture of ingredients. Addition of ingredients such as salt, sugar, and silica can help adjust the final water activity to a desired endpoint.

An intermediate food is considered safe with regard to pathogen contamination, but is subject to spoilage organisms, enzymatic and non-enzymatic breakdown and physical changes. The US Code of Federal Regulations (21 CFR 110.80 (14)) states that intermediate foods that rely on the control of water activity for preventing growth of undesirable microorganisms shall be processed to, and maintained at, a safe moisture level. Monitoring water activity, adjusting the soluble solids:water ratio or controlling packaging can accomplish this. Further drying, or use of solutes such as salt, sucrose or sorbitol could be used to lower the water activity; however this might not produce the desired final product characteristics. Preservatives such as sodium benzoate, propionic acid and potassium sorbate can be used to control microbial growth. Factors such as pH, target microorganisms, taste and cost can be used to decide on the appropriate preservative. Water isotherms should be used to predict the physical stability of the product, taking critical limits for desired characteristics into account.

High moisture foods (> 0.85 Aw), such as canned pet foods, must be processed in conformance with low acid canned food regulations (21 CFR, Part 113). These regulations state that critical factors such as water activity must be used in conjunction with thermal processing.

Conclusion

In order to produce a pet food that is both commercially viable and safe, water activity must be used as both a development tool and a quality assurance mechanism. Water activity values are an extremely important consideration in any type of pet food, since water activity plays a role in the physical, chemical and biological stability of the product. Several methods have been given for evaluating and determining the effect of water activity on a particular formula. The challenge to the pet food industry is to use the right combination of ingredients, processing and packaging to create products that meet safety and quality standards, meet cost parameters and still maintain integrity of design to satisfy consumers.

References

Decagon. (2003). Water activity and pet foods. *Water Activity News*, p. 6.

Fontana, A.J. (2000). Water activity's role in food safety and quality. Decagon Application notes. http://www.decagon.com.

Gock, M.A., A.D. Hocking, J.I. Pitt and P.G. Poulos. (2003). Influence of temperature, water activity and pH on growth of some xerophilic fungi. *Int. J. Food Microbiol.* **81(1)**: 11-9.

Lowe, J.A. and S.J. Kershaw. (1995). Water activity-moisture content relationship as a predictive indicator for control of spoilage in commercial pet diet components. *Anim. Feed Sci. Tech.* **56**: 187-194.

Salwin, H. (1963). Moisture levels required for stability in dehydrated foods. **Food Tech**. **17**: 1114-1121.

Scudamore, K.A., M.T. Hetmanski, S. Nawax, J. Naylor and S. Rainbird. (1997). Determination of mycotoxins in pet foods sold for domestic pets and wild birds using linked column immunoassay cleanup and HPLC. *Food Addit. Contam.* **14(2)**: 175-86.

US Food and Drug Administration. (2005). Code of Federal Regulations, *CFR 21*, Part 110. Washington, DC.

Effects of mycotoxins in domestic pet species

Josef Böhm

Fungi are ubiquitous in the environment, and are common contaminants of raw materials, such as cereal grains, used in animal feed. Many different types of mycotoxins have been classified, and are formed as secondary metabolites from fungi including *Fusarium, Aspergillus, Claviceps* and *Penicillium* species. All animals are known to be susceptible to these toxins, although symptoms may vary between species.

Domestic pets are defined as those animals commonly cared for within households, and include cats, dogs, ornamental birds, rabbits, guinea pigs, but not horses, mice or rats. Over the last decade, the importance of domestic pets in developed countries has grown dramatically. Taking the European Union as an example, in Austria, cats are found in more than 28% of households, dogs in 16%, ornamental birds in 5%, aquarium fish in 4%, rabbits in 2.5%, guinea pigs in 2%, and hamsters and turtles in 1% of households (Statist. Zentralamt, 2001).

The adverse effects of fungal toxins have been well documented in many species of animals, particularly farm animals. However, only a few papers address mycotoxicosis in pets. Puschner (2002) reviewed the clinical and pathological effects of some mycotoxins on pets. In addition, Devegowda (2000) and Bird (2000) have examined the relevance of mycotoxins in pet foods. This general lack of information makes it difficult to assess the relevance of mycotoxins to pet health. Descriptions of food-induced symptoms have been reported in cases of the ingestion of aflatoxins, tremorgens (penitrem A and roquefortine) and ochratoxins in dogs. Experimentally, the effects of trichothecenes, patulin, penicillic acid, and cyclopiazonic acid have been studied in dogs and cats.

For the most toxic compounds maximum regulatory limits in the European Union have been defined. For aflatoxin B_1 this is 10 μg/kg in complete feedstuffs (Council Directive 1999/29/EC). The US

169

Food and Drug Administration has only established an 'action' level (FDA Regulatory Guidance for Toxins and Contaminants) of 20 ppb for corn, peanut products, cottonseed meal, and other animal feeds and feed ingredients.

Although there is less research into the effects of mycotoxicosis in companion animal species, they are still severely affected by these toxins. Suspected cases of aflatoxicosis in dogs were reported in the USA during 2003 and 2005, when more than 100 dogs died as a direct consequence. Pet food was identified as the causal agent, and the manufacturer issued a recall of several products made at a plant in South Carolina (Muirhead, 2006; Stenske *et al.*, 2006). The European Commission was also informed (RASFF, 2006). Such incidences highlight the importance of raw material quality control in pet food manufacturing.

Aflatoxins

Aflatoxins are toxic secondary metabolites of *Aspergillus* spp., such as *A. parasiticus* and *A. flavus*. Aflatoxins cause disease symptoms in livestock, domestic animals, and humans throughout the world. Due to their high toxicity and carcinogenic properties, aflatoxins have probably received greater research and monitoring attention than other mycotoxins. In the early 1960's, when more than 100,000 young turkeys in England died as the result of an apparently new disease (later named 'Turkey X disease'), aflatoxicosis was found to be the cause of death.

In the 1950's, before 'Turkey X disease' was reported; epizootics of fatal hepatitis in dogs were diagnosed provisionally as 'hepatitis X' (Seibold and Bailey, 1952; Seibold, 1953; Newberne *et al.* 1955). At that time, the aetiology was unknown; however, lesions were similar to those observed in the mouldy corn poisoning of swine (Bailey and Groth, 1959), and also resembled lesions found in animals with confirmed aflatoxicosis. After isolation and characterisation of the toxins produced by *A. flavus*, a causal connection was made between aflatoxicosis and hepatitis X.

Subsequent experimental studies have proven that dogs are susceptible to hepatic damage due to aflatoxins (Newberne *et al.* 1966). In addition to hepatitis and sudden death, symptoms of acute aflatoxicosis in both dogs and cats include vomiting, depression, polydipsia, and polyuria. Rabbits show the greatest sensitivity to aflatoxins, with LD_{50} levels of only 0.4 mg/kg body weight. In experiments with dogs, death usually occurs within 3 days of exposure, and LD_{50} levels range from 0.5 to 1.0 mg/kg body weight. In cats, the LD_{50} varies between 0.3 to 0.6 mg/kg body weight, depending on the age of the animal (Patterson, 1977). Pathological examinations of affected animals revealed enlarged livers, disseminated intravascular coagulation, and internal haemorrhaging. In sub-acute aflatoxicosis (0.5 – 1 mg/kg pet food administered over 2-3 weeks) dogs and cats became lethargic, anorexic, and jaundiced. This is occasionally followed by disseminated intravascular coagulation and death. In chronic aflatoxicosis (as defined by doses of 0.05 – 0.3 mg/kg of pet food administered over 6-8 weeks) dogs and cats showed clinical signs similar to those for the sub-acute phase, but jaundice was the predominant manifestation. Histopathology of animals with chronic aflatoxicosis revealed shrunken livers with extensive fibrosis, correlating with the hepatotoxic effects of aflatoxins observed in many animal species.

Frequently observed clinical signs of experimentally induced aflatoxicosis in dogs include anorexia, followed by dehydration, somnolence, and jaundice. Gross pathological changes included sub-serosal and sub-mucosal petechial haemorrhages throughout the thoracic and peritoneal cavities, and yellow, mottled livers. Necrosis and petechial haemorrhages in the gall-bladder, pancreas, kidneys, thymus, heart, and adrenal glands have also been described. Microscopically, acute hepatitis (characterised by fatty degeneration and hepatic cell necrosis), bile duct proliferation, fibrosis, and hepatic cell regeneration have also been observed (Edds, 1973).

Natural outbreaks of aflatoxicosis – reported cases in dogs

There have been reports of outbreaks of chronic liver disease in packs of dogs kennelled together (Greene et al.,1977), where anorexia, depression, polyuria, polydipsia, icterus and a terminal haemorrhagic diathesis were observed. Thrombocytopenia, hypofibrinogenemia, elevated fibrinogen degradation metabolites, prolonged activated partial thromboplastin times, and one-stage prothrombin times were associated with haemorrhagic crises. Aflatoxicosis was confirmed by the presence of significant levels of aflatoxin B in the commercial dog food being fed. In addition, sub-acute hepatitis was found on necropsy.

Liggett et al. (1986) published case descriptions of high morbidity and mortality in hunting dogs. Clinical signs included icterus, anorexia, and listlessness. Additional laboratory examinations revealed toxic hepatitis, bilirubinuria, and anaemia. The diagnosis was confirmed by the analysis of aflatoxin B_1 in tissues. A second case, involving a dead Beagle that had been fed a ration containing cornmeal contaminated with 511 ng/g aflatoxin B_1 and B_2, was also reported.

A natural outbreak of aflatoxicosis was observed in 10 dogs in the Republic of South Africa (Bastianello *et al.*, 1987), with 1 acute case, 7 sub-acute cases and 2 chronic cases within the affected pack. These were classified on the basis of the nature, degree, and extent of the following histopathology: hepatocellular fatty degeneration, necrosis or regeneration; proliferation of bile ductules; accumulation of bile within the canaliculi; fibroplasias; mucoid degeneration, necrosis or segmental atrophy of the larger intrahepatic bile ducts.

Fatty degeneration was noted in the livers of all ten cases, and bile stasis was seen in four dogs. Varying degrees of fibrosis were present, depending on the stage of the disease. In the two chronic cases, in which nodular regeneration was observed, fibrosis was pronounced. Other macroscopic findings included icterus, anaemia, ascites, hydrothorax, hydropericardium, anasarca, pulmonary oedema, gastro-enterorhagia, and nephrosis.

Bingham, Phillips and Bauer (2003) reported an episode in Texas in 1998, where 17 brands of commercial food formulated for dogs were contaminated with aflatoxin B_1, with levels ranging from 150 and 300 ppb. Fifty-five dogs died from eating the contaminated food, but it is likely that many more went unreported. The most affected animals had eaten the contaminated diet for at least 90 and up to 120 days. Hot spots of aflatoxin concentrations in a batch of corn were identified, as the consignment had not been incorporated into standard samples used for quality control. This is a major issue for feed and food manufacturers, as sampling raw materials for mycotoxins is fraught with problems because fungal growth tends to be in focal 'clumps'.

When high aflatoxin levels in corn are evident in such cases, a second line of defence may have negated the effects of the toxins. It is known that certain commercially developed products can bind and negate the toxin effects of mycotoxins in feed. Hydrated sodium calcium aluminosilicate (HSCAS) and specialist yeast cell wall fractions (Mycosorb™) can reduce the absorption of aflatoxins in the gut of animals. These products sequester and immobilise aflatoxins in the gastrointestinal tract, thus reducing the bio-availability of aflatoxins in a dose-dependent manner. HSCAS is a structured clay and is used as an anti-caking commercial feed additive, whereas Mycosorb is a carbohydrate-based product with a large, adsorbent surface area. It is recommended that 5 kg/t of HSCAS, or 1 kg/t Mycosorb™, is mixed into the diet to ensure protection against toxicity. Bingham *et al.*, (2004) demonstrated that dogs fed pet food contaminated with aflatoxin had significantly lower levels of metabolites in urine when HSCAS was fed in the diet.

Diet-associated hepatic failure and immune-mediated haemolytic anaemia have been reported in a Weimaraner dog (Smith *et al.*, 2005), however in this case it was not possible to determine the exact cause. The dog was clinically treated, even though the cause of its presenting symptoms remained unclear. The diet manufacturer initiated a voluntary recall on the commercial food the animal was receiving in case the symptoms were related to contaminated raw materials.

Stenske *et al.*, (2006) have documented in detail the multiple cases of aflatoxicosis in the USA that occurred in 2005. Analyses conducted by the FDA confirmed aflatoxin contamination, resulting in a recall of 19 products manufactured at a single plant in South Carolina. Recall instructions advised pet owners to discontinue feeding the product and to return unused food to their retailer. Concerned pet owners were instructed to consult a veterinarian if their dog had clinical signs that included loss of appetite, yellow coloration of white skin and eyes, severe vomiting combined with bloody diarrhoea, discoloured urine, and fever. This highlights the need for rapid recognition of the adverse effects involving consumption of contaminated foods, and the need to communicate effectively with the appropriate groups involved (e.g. retailers, manufacturers, regulatory agencies, pet owners and veterinarians). It is important, under these circumstances, to retain food samples, product labels, and biological samples to aid in the identification of contaminated foods.

In a review of mycotoxicosis in pets, Rumbeiha (2003) stated that mycotoxin contamination, although rare, is ruthless. Studies have almost exclusively addressed individual, often purified, mycotoxins, ignoring the real field conditions where multiple mycotoxins are co-produced by moulds. Several chronological aflatoxicosis cases in dogs fed 50-300 ppb aflatoxin B1 over a period of 6-8 weeks have been shown to cause chronic symptoms. Ingestion of low amounts of aflatoxin in food (20-100ppb) may also cause immunosuppression, rendering the animal unable to respond to regular vaccinations. Cancer is a long-term effect of aflatoxin exposure.

The high morbidity and mortality rate associated with outbreaks of aflatoxicosis and the failure of dogs to respond to symptomatic treatment often prompts practitioners to refer dogs or submit tissue specimens to veterinary hospitals and diagnostic laboratories. An immediate ration change is indicated in most cases of toxic hepatitis, pending analysis of the food.

In contrast, no natural outbreaks of aflatoxicosis have been reported in cats. This may be due to the fact that cat food rations contain mainly meat and meat products (approximately 70%) and lower amounts of cereals (approximately 30%). As cereals are at much higher risk of contamination than meat (unless taken from an animal exposed to mycotoxins, which may then accumulate in certain organs such as the liver), the increased reliance on cereals in pet food formulations has increased the risk of exposure to toxins and the development of mycotoxicosis in pets.

The introduction of strict quality control and quality assurance of incoming material in the pet food industry, and the development of accurate screening methods for animal food in recent years has led to a vast reduction in the amounts of aflatoxin B_1 in pet food. Consequently, there have been only occasional reports of aflatoxicosis in dogs recently.

Aflatoxin occurrence in pet foods

Analysis of 35 samples of dog and cat foods in Mexico, using immuno-affinity columns and HPLC (Sharma and Marquez, 2001) identified maize as the common ingredient in contaminated samples. Aflatoxin B_1 was found with the highest frequency and was present at particularly high levels (72 und 60 ng/g) in six samples (17 %) of both dog and cat food.

The mycofloral species in commercial dry pet foods has been examined in research conducted in Argentina (Bueno *et al.*, 2001). Ten fungal genera and one fungus (classified as *Mycelia sterilia*) were identified. Predominant genera included *Aspergillus* (62%), *Rhizopus* (48%), and *Mucor* (38%). The most common among *Aspergillus* was *A. flavus* followed by *A. niger*, and *A. terreus*. *Mucor racemosus* was followed, in frequency of occurrence, by *M. plumbus* and *M. globosus*. Certain genera and species isolated and identified from these foods are potential mycotoxin producers, and represent a risk for companion animal health. A particularly important practice for minimizing fungal growth is maintaining the moisture content of raw materials and food below 10%.

The occurrence of aflatoxins in Brazilian pet foods (dog, cat and bird foods) was reported by Maia and Bastos de Siqueira (2002), who found aflatoxin in 12% of the samples analysed. Of 45 dog foods 7 % tested positive for aflatoxins. Of 25 cat foods 4 % were positive and of 30 bird foods 27 % were positive. Levels detected varied between 15 and 374 µg/kg, and all pet foods formulated with peanuts scored positive for aflatoxin B_1. Such levels of aflatoxins pose a risk to animal health, especially in bird food. Aflatoxin concentrations in dog and cat food were lower, because corn, rice, soybean and wheat were the main ingredients and peanuts were not included in the diet.

Basalan *et al.* (2004) analysed pelleted dog food and found 7 ppb aflatoxin B$_1$ with 100 % incidence of contamination in 21 tested samples. In a survey of aflatoxin concentrations in wild bird seed purchased in Texas, Henke *et al.* (2001) suggested that feeding wildlife may contribute to their exposure to aflatoxins. Bags of wild bird seed (n = 142) were purchased from grain co-operatives, grocery stores, and pet shops located in Texas during the spring and summer of 1999. Aflatoxin concentrations ranged from non-detectable levels to 2780 μg/kg, with 17% of samples having aflatoxin concentrations greater than 100 μg/kg. High contamination appeared to be a consequence of formulating using corn as the ingredient. Using such feeds exposes granivorous songbirds to aflatoxin and may contribute significantly to their morbidity and mortality.

Ochratoxin A

Ochratoxin A (OTA) is an important compound because of its high toxicity. It is a potent nephrotoxic (i.e. specifically affects the kidneys) secondary metabolite produced by moulds such as *Aspergillus ochraceus* and *Penicillium verrucosum*. Ochratoxin A is widely distributed in Europe and North America and has been identified as a natural contaminant of agricultural commodities, apparently causing porcine nephropathy following degradation of the proximal tubules and interstitial fibroses (Blank *et al.*, 1999; Krogh, 1992).

Young Beagle dogs been shown to be very sensitive to OTA. A daily oral dose of between 0.2 and 0.3 mg/kg body weight was found to be deadly within 10 to 14 days of continued ingestion (Szczech *et al.*, 1973a; 1973b; 1974). Clinical signs observed at this dose level include loss of appetite, vomiting, tenesmus, increased body temperature, tonsillitis, bloody and viscous faeces, polydipsia, polyuria, dehydration, paralysis, and death.

Pathological disturbances due to ochratoxicosis are generally associated with kidney damage, for example the specific weight of urine may be reduced. In addition, cell counts in the sediment, protein and glucose levels, and the activities of lactate dehydrogenase, leucinaminopeptidase, glutamate pyruvate transaminase, and alkaline phosphatase may all be increased, although serum enzyme activities were unaltered. Serum sodium and potassium levels may be reduced as a consequence of OTA exposure, whereas secondary dehydration, haemoglobin concentration, total blood protein, and haematocrit can be increased. Gross dissections revealed pale brownish kidneys, hyperemic tonsils, and viscous bloody enteritis of the distal ileum, caecum, colon, and rectum. Additional oedemas and hyperemic and partial necrotic lymph nodes, with necrosis and desquamation of epithelial cells from the proximal renal tubules was also observed. Ultra-structural changes, such as proliferation and dilation of the endoplasmic reticulum of the proximal epithelial tubuli cells may be evident.

In a study conducted by Kitchen *et al.* (1977a; 1977b), dogs were observed pacing and vomiting when receiving an OTA dose of 0.2 mg/kg. At higher doses (between 0.2 and 3.0 mg/kg) symptoms included anorexia, polydipsia, polyuria, anxiety, prostration, and death. Necropsy findings included epithelial degeneration (proximal tubules), mucohaemorrhagic enteritis (caecum, colon, and rectum), and necrosis of the lymphoid tissues (spleen, tonsil, thymus, and peripheral lymph nodes). When OTA was ingested alone or in combination with citrinin by young Beagle dogs for 2 weeks, the symptoms observed were similar to those described above. However in those receiving combined mycotoxins, mortality rate was much higher and clinical signs were more dramatic, indicating a synergistic toxic effect. Such synergies have been well documented in other species.

Gareis *et al.*, (1987) reported a case of 'fading puppy' syndrome in Afghan puppies following ingestion of ochratoxin A-contaminated milk powder. Clinical signs appeared a few hours after the first food using the affected powder. Pathological and histological findings suggested canine herpes virus as the most probably cause of the syndrome, but an association between the intake of low levels of OTA contaminated food, a possible dysbiosis and the manifestation of the multi-causal viral infection was also hypothesised.

The occurrence of OTA in pet foods

Studies regarding the contamination of petfood with OTA have been published. Twenty-six canned and 17 dry pet foods for cats and dogs; along with 26 feline kidney samples (with and without pathological changes) were surveyed for OTA residues by Razzazi-Fazeli *et al.* (2001). Analysis of OTA was carried out by an isocratic HPLC system, based on reverse phase with fluorescence detection. Ochratoxin A was detected in 47% of the pet food samples, although those that were positive, generally contained low amounts of OTA (0.1 – 0.8 μg/kg pet food). Higher levels were only detected in two pet food samples (3.2 and 13.1 μg/kg). Low concentrations of OTA was found in cat kidneys, 16 of which were positive, with concentration levels ranging between 0.35 and 1.5 μg/kg tissue.

Pühringer (2003) investigated 101 feline kidneys, both with and without pathological alterations, and determined the OTA residue present. Thirty-nine kidneys were OTA positive, and minor OTA contamination, in the range of 0.11 to 0.3 μg/kg, was identified in 23 cases. In the remaining 16 samples, OTA ranged from 0.31 to 5.18 μg/kg. No significant correlation was found between the levels of OTA in feline kidneys and any pathological changes.

The contamination of cat food was analysed, using 55 commercial samples, of which 45 were canned and 10 dry products. Fourteen cat foods tested positive for OTA, with values in the range 0.11 to 2.17 μg/kg. Seven of canned and seven of the dry pet food samples tested positive for OTA.

In dog foods, seven out of 29 dry food samples and two out of 11 wet foods were contaminated with between 7 – 40 and 54-115 ppb, with a detection limit of 1.9 ppb (Songsermsakul et al., 2004). The OTA positive dry food samples were additionally contaminated with DON.

Fusarium mycotoxins

Trichothecenes

While aflatoxins are undoubtedly the most hepatotoxic, *Fusarium* toxins have recently been given more attention (Böhm, 2000 a, b; Placinta et al, 1999) as they are considerably more widespread, and are found to contaminate grain and produce toxins even in what has previously been considered 'safer' temperate climates. In Europe, infection of agricultural crops with *Fusarium* spp. is a major concern (Razzazi-Fazeli et al. 2003). Factors such as temperature, rain fall, and the type of host plant influence the distribution of *Fusarium* spp. in cereals. *Fusarium* causes 'head blight' and *Giberella* 'ear rot' in cereals, two diseases that have important economic consequences in arable farming.

Trichothecenes (TCT) are secondary metabolites of *Fusarium* moulds, and a major contaminant of cereal crops. TCT are often found in cereals such as maize, barley, wheat, and oats that have been grown in regions with temperate climates. Commercial dry pet foods may contain large amounts of TCT if formulated with contaminated grain or cereal by-products. TCTs can be divided into sub-classes based on their chemical structure. Ingestion may lead to weight loss, decreased food conversion, food refusal and vomiting. TCTs can inhibit protein synthesis and have immunosuppressive effects. A-type trichothecenes are more toxic than B-type trichothecenes, since they have a dermotoxic effect, leading to necrosis and haemorrhage of tissue that have been exposed to contact.

The most important trichothecenes are deoxynivalenol (DON), which is sometimes referred to as vomitoxin, nivalenol (NIV), T-2 toxin, and diacetoxyscirpenol (DAS). B-trichothecenes such as deoxynivalenol (DON) mainly cause food refusal and vomiting (Canady *et al.*, 2002). Toxin stability is of particular concern because DON is known to be stable under processing conditions such as sterilisation at 120°C (Hughes *et al*, 1999) autoclaving, or extrusion cooking (Wolf-Hall *et al*, 1999).

Type A-TCT's, such as T-2 toxin and DAS, have extremely toxic effects on skin and mucous surfaces and induce lesions on the mucosa of the mouth and oesophageal region of poultry and pigs. The most toxic trichothecene is T-2 toxin, which causes dermatitis of the nose and buccal commissures in pigs. The immuno-toxicity of type A-TCT, especially that of T-2 toxin, is less immuno-toxic than the type B-TCT (Hussein and Brasel 2001).

Lutsky and Mor (1981) have shown that exposure of cats to T-2 toxin results in chronic lethal intoxication, characterized by pancytopenia, haemorrhagic diatheses, bone marrow aplasia, diminished haemostasis, severe lymphatic tissue alterations, and histopathological changes in proliferative tissues. Clinical signs included vomiting, bloody faeces, weakness, lassitude, ataxia, dyspnea, dehydration, loss of weight, and pre-terminal anorexia. The gross and microscopic tissue changes seen in affected cats were similar to alimentary toxic aleukia, a frequently fatal mycotoxin-induced disease in humans.

Observations in dogs exposed to 0.5 mg/kg body weight DAS (Coppock *et al.*, 1989) showed moderate to severe necrosis of bone marrow haematopoietic elements. Sequential increases in the type and number of abnormal cells in the blood was noted, suggesting a successive destruction of haematopoietic elements. A marked shift in the neutrophil population was found in animals exposed to DAS, with metarubricytes and large platelets found in blood, and lymphocytes replaced with immature cells. Pigs appear to be more sensitive to DAS than dogs, which in turn are more sensitive than cattle. Residue studies of DAS and rapid recovery after exposure suggest that DAS is metabolised and excreted.

DON and other trichothecenes are highly toxic to animals if ingested in contaminated feed, and can cause sub-lethal toxicosis in lower doses, where clinical effects such as reduced weight gain, emesis, and diarrhoea are observed. Inhibition of protein synthesis appears to be the main mechanism of toxicity, resulting in cell death. Acute signs include gastrointestinal haemorrhage, with vomiting; weight loss and loss of appetite being chronic sequelae.

There are no specific gross or histological lesions associated with TCT mycotoxicosis. Exposure can only be confirmed by the detection of TCT mycotoxins in suspected food. Hughes et al. (1999) conducted trials examining DON exposure in dogs and cats, from which they calculated the amounts of DON required in food to produce toxicity symptoms (vomiting and reduced food intake). Food intake was significantly reduced at concentrations of 4.5 mg/kg food. Naturally contaminated wheat, containing DON at 37 mg/kg and 1mg/kg of 15-acetylDON was present in the pet food formulations, giving 0, 1, 2, 4, 6, 8, and 10 mg of DON/kg. No other *Fusarium* toxins were detected in these diets, and DON was found to be stable during conventional extrusion processing used to manufacture these pet foods. Dogs previously exposed to DON-contaminated food were able to preferentially select uncontaminated food. Food intake was significantly reduced by DON concentrations greater than 4.5 mg/kg, and vomiting was observed at levels of 8 and 10 mg/kg food. When the same researchers (Hughes et al., 1999) fed the similarly contaminated wheat to groups of mature American shorthair cats (1-9 years old) for 14 days, food intake was significantly reduced when it contained DON exceeding 7.7 mg/kg (equivalent to 0.38 mg/kg body weight per day).

The occurrence of DON in 40 dog foods (29 kibble food and 11 canned food) from Austrian and German retail stores has been reported (Songsermsakul et al., 2004). Dry food samples were found to be contaminated with between 22 – 1837 ppb DON, with 8 canned foods being below the detection limit (19 ppb). The higher concentration of DON in dry food is probably due to its higher cereal content in comparison with canned food. Seven out of 29 dry food were also contaminated with OTA.

Leung and Smith (2006b) studied the effects of blended grains (corn and wheat) naturally contaminated with *Fusarium* mycotoxins (4 ppm) on the health of mature Beagle dogs. Dogs exposed to contaminated food during a 7 day challenge period showed a significant decrease in food intake and a slight decrease in body weight. It was concluded that feeding grains naturally contaminated with lower levels of multiple *Fusarium* toxins (DON, 15acetyl-DON and zearalenone) was not toxic enough to induce vomiting, however watery faeces were also observed in the exposed animals, suggesting that low-level Fusarium mycotoxicosis can lead to gastric disturbances. Providing non-contaminated food resulted in a rapid recovery.

Zearalenone

Zearalenone (ZEA) is a secondary fungal metabolite of *Fusarium* and has been shown to have hormonal (oestrogen analogue) activities. Pigs are especially sensitive to this mycotoxin, showing clinical signs of hyper-oestrogenism, which is associated with severe reproductive disorders. Oestrogenic effects with ZEA also have been reported in other species, including guinea-pigs and rabbits (Mirocha *et al*. 1968). In dogs, a reduced number of corpus lutea were found following 13 weeks of exposure to a diet containing ZEA where ingestion was 1 mg/kg body weight per day (Hidy *et al*. 1977). Zwierzchovski *et al*. (2004) considered the occurrence of zearalenone and its derivates in both standard and therapeutic foods formulated for companion animals. Eighty-four percent of the 57 samples tested were positive for zearalenone, with a maximum contamination level of 300 ppb. Breeders should expect issues in reproductive performance in bitches exposed to these levels of toxins.

Tremorgenic mycotoxins

Tremorgenic mycotoxins have indole alkaloid characteristics, and are produced by different genera of *Penicillium*, *Aspergillus*, and *Claviceps* (Cole, 1981; Cole and Dorner, 1985).The main toxic effects include changes in the central nervous system (Schell, 2000). Sources of these mycotoxins include dairy foods, walnuts or peanuts, stored grains, and spaghetti, which all may be used as raw materials in pet food. A two-year observational study at the Animal Poison Control Centre (APCC) into the incidence of tremorgenic mycotoxins revealed 25 suspected cases.

Penitrem A and roquefortine, two of the most important tremorgenic mycotoxins, have been linked to natural disease outbreaks in small animals. Various *Penicillium* spp., including *P. crustosum*, *P. roqueforti*, and *P. cyclopium*, may potentially produce tremorgenic mycotoxins and have been isolated from mouldy cream cheese and other foodstuffs (Richard and Arp, 1979, Hocking *et al*, 1988, Richard *et al*, 1981, Kokkonen *et al*, 2005). An important producer of the toxin roquefortine is *Penicillium roqueforti*, which is found primarily in blue cheese (Ware *et al*, 1980). Acute muscle tremors, seizures, and prostration are typical clinical symptoms, and several hypothetical mechanisms of action have been proposed for penitrem A toxicosis. The severity of the clinical and pathologic features of this toxin in dogs is dose dependent, with mildly affected dogs displaying transitory muscle tremors and ataxia lasting 2 to 4 hours. Higher doses can cause death during seizures, but a progressive return to normal neurological function can occur after 1 or 2 days. Visceral petechial haemorrhages, liver necrosis, and hyperthermia have also been observed in animals exposed to contaminated food. Penitrem A and roquefortine are absorbed in the gut and excreted through the bile (Wilson and Payne, 1994), and enterohepatic re-circulation and continued re-absorption are known to contribute to the prolonged period of time required for recovery.

Penitrem A toxicosis in dogs typically appears within half an hour of toxin ingestion. Clinical symptoms have been described by Hocking et al. (1988) and Lowes et al. (1992), and include weakness, muscle tremors, increased irritability, rigidity, hyperactivity, and occasionally fever. Exhaustion may follow the increased muscle activity; elevated serum aspartate aminotransferase, increased creatine kinase, hyperthermia, rhabdomyelosis, and dehydration also can be seen. Often vomiting is observed before the onset of neurological symptoms.

Penitrem A has various toxic physiological mechanisms. It is a lipophilic (fat soluble) molecule, a property that enables it to cross the blood-brain barrier, and influence the release of acetylcholine, and important neurotransmitter (Wilson et al, 1972). Cole and Cox (1981) showed that the toxin can antagonize glycine production, which is an important amino acid required for growth and various metabolic activities, and can substitute for γ-aminobutyric acid (Selala et al., 1989).

Diagnosis can be established after the exclusion of other tremorgenic agents, such as strychnine, metaldehyde, bromethaline, organophosphorus compounds, carbamates, methylxanthines, pyrethroids, and chlorinated hydrocarbons. Penitrem A or roquefortine can be isolated from samples of vomit, gastric lavage washings, stomach contents, or bile (Braselton and Rumler, 1996; Lowes et al, 1992). Treatments include provoked emesis and gastric lavage, performed under anaesthesia. As with other intoxications, activated charcoal can be administered orally to bind the toxin. Additionally, sodium bicarbonate administration is recommended if an acid-base imbalance has occurred. Diazepam is the treatment of choice followed by barbiturates (Lowes et al, 1992, Richard et al, 1981), as sedatives and anaesthetics can reduce symptoms and allow recovery.

Although a specific antidote is not available for penitrem A, pentobarbital has been used to control seizures and excessive motor activity. Fluid therapy and short-duration corticosteroids may counteract shock and stabilise lysosomal membranes. Hyperthermia (fever) associated with the acute neurological syndrome can be controlled by sedation and cold water baths. Supportive care and close monitoring is emphasised to prohibit any aspiration pneumonia. *Penicillium* and *Aspergillus* species are the fungi most frequently isolated from refrigerators and mouldy foodstuffs in the home, and care should be taken in disposal of contaminated garbage.

Intra-peritoneal administered doses of 0.5 mg /kg penitrem A have been shown to cause acute tremors and death in dogs (Hayes *et al.*, 1976), with symptoms developing within 30 minutes when exposed to 0.13 mg of penitrem A. At lower doses, however, the animals recovered completely. Severe muscle tremors in dogs have been reported following an oral dose of 0.18 mg/kg body weight.

Several cases of natural exposure to this toxin have been published. Arp and Richard (1979) reported a case of intoxication of two Australian Shepherd dogs that had eaten mouldy cream cheese, infected with dark blue-green *Penicillium crustosum*. Experimental mice and a Beagle dog fed the same contaminated sample showed similar tremorgenic symptoms as the two affected dogs, thereby identifying penitrem A as the causal agent. Puls and Ladyman (1988) described intoxication of an eight-year-old Fox terrier cross Pekingese male dog, displaying shivering, moderate tetanic spasms and mild opisthotonus. A tentative diagnosis of strychnine poisoning was made. Toxicological analysis revealed the presence of roquefortine in mouldy blue cheese that the dog had eaten.

In the case of a 1-year-old Siberian Husky presenting symptoms of severe muscle tremors after consuming a mouldy hamburger bun (Hocking *et al.*, 1988), *P. crustosum* and penitrem A toxin were isolated from the remaining portion of the bun. When grown in pure culture, the isolated *P. crustosum* produced large amounts of penitrem A, along with other penitrem compounds. In Canada, a Labrador retriever was poisoned after consuming garbage (Walter 2002), and showed symptoms including polypnea, tachycardia and ataxia. Penitrem A and roquefortine were diagnosed, and removal of the mycotoxins from the stomach allowed the dog to recover within a few days.

In South Africa, mouldy rice contaminated with *Penicillium crustosum* eaten by dogs induced a tremorgenic neuro-mycotoxicosis (Naude *et al*, 2002), resulting in vomiting, tremor and ataxia. Vomit analysis yielded penitrem A and roquefortine and was confirmed by LC-MS. The dogs recovered after treatment with anaesthetics.

Four dogs in Massachusetts were reportedly affected by tremorgenic mycotoxins (Boysen et al, 2002), after penitrem A and roquefortine were found in stomach contents. Treatments included reducing the absorption of the mycotoxins from the gastrointestinal tract (by binding the toxins) and control of the tremors and seizures by sedatives and anaesthetics. Two dogs from Iowa became intoxicated with penitrem A and roquefortine (Young et al, 2003) after eating mouldy dairy products retrieved from the household garbage. The clinical symptoms again resembled strychnine poisoning, however roquefortine was determined as the predominant toxin in a mouldy cream cheese wrapper, and penitrem A was detected in discarded macaroni and cheese garbage.

Cyclopiazonic acid

Another mycotoxin produced by *Aspergillus flavus*, known as cyclopiazonic acid (CPA), may adversely affect dogs if ingested. Sub-acute toxic effects of orally administered CPA have been characterized in dogs by Nuehring et al. (1985), where animals were exposed to doses ranging between 0.05, 0.25, 0.5 and 1.0 mg/kg of body weight for 90 days. All dogs receiving the high dose groups died. Clinical signs of intoxication appeared between 2 and 44 days after exposure and included anorexia, vomiting, diarrhoea, pyrexia, dehydration, weight loss, and loss of CNS function. The entire alimentary tract exhibited diffuse hyperaemia, with focal areas of haemorrhage and ulceration. Other lesions included renal infarcts, necrotising epididymitis, and ulcerative dermatitis, and microscopic lesions, including ulceration, necrosis, vasculitis, lymphoid necrosis, karyomegaly in several organs, and decreased mitotic activity of the intestinal crypt epithelium. Ulcerative and necrotic damage was usually associated with vascular lesions. Pathological changes included leukocytosis, neutrophilia, lymphopenia, monocytosis, and increased serum alkaline phosphatase activity.

Patulin and penicillic acid

Patulin and penicillic acid are produced by *Penicillium* and *Aspergillus* spp., often found in mouldy feeds and cheeses. Patulin is also present in rotten fruits, apple juice, and mouldy bread. The toxicity of patulin, and the interaction between patulin and penicillic acid in dogs, have been studied by Reddy et al. (1979). The most sensitive organs were found to be the lungs and gastrointestinal tract. Clinical signs of toxicosis included haematemesis, diarrhoea, lethargy, pulmonary haemorrhage and pulmonary oedema when patulin was administered intravenously at doses greater than 10 mg/kg of body weight. Dogs that received 10 mg/kg body weight penicillic acid on its own showed slight inappetence, but no other clinical signs, indicating a synergistic interaction between patulin and penicillic acid.

Ergot alkaloids

The fungus *Claviceps purpurea* produces three important toxic alkaloids, namely ergotine, ergotamine and ergotoxin. They may be present in all grain types, but are especially found to contaminate triticale, rye and wheat. Toxicity is mediated via vasoconstriction and thrombosis in peripheral capillaries, and can result in severe damage to extremities. Chronic intoxication is more likely to produce neuronal symptoms including tremors and seizures.

Wolter and Jean (1997) have described dietary intoxications with ergot alkaloids in domestic carnivores, and suggest that these alkaloids are important contributors to feline dysautonomia. Symptoms include acute peripheral vasoconstriction (extending to gangrene), disseminated coagulation, haemorrhage, and female reproductive disorders including agalactia. Chronic intoxication produces neurological symptoms, such as hyper-excitation and tremors, combined with ataxia. Toxic effects are observed when ergot inclusion exceeds 1 g/kg food. Quantitative determination of ergot alkaloids in foods poses analytical problems, however if the fungus is separated from the grains, the task is easier (Mellor, 2003).

Multiple mycotoxin contamination in pet foods

Scudamore *et al.* (1997) analysed over 100 samples of pet foods for the presence of mycotoxins, including 35 samples of cereal-based dog and cat foods, 15 samples of domestic bird seeds, and 15 samples of wild bird food. All samples were examined for aflatoxins B_1, B_2, G_1, G_2 and ochratoxin A, 20 samples were analysed for fumonisins B_1 and B_2. Of the 100 samples eighty-four percent contained no measurable concentrations of mycotoxins. Low levels of aflatoxin B_1 were found in one sample of cat food, and 370 μg/kg aflatoxin B_1 was found in one sample of peanuts marketed for wild birds. Ochratoxin A was detected in 10% of all samples, but in low concentrations; the highest concentration (7 μg/kg) occurring in a sample of pet bird food. Fumonisins were found in 30% of the 20 samples tested, with a maximum of 750 μg/kg total fumonisins found in a sample of cat food. The significance of fumonisin contamination is uncertain at present. Five samples each of dog and cat food were analysed for mould count and fungal species. After storage under controlled simulated damp conditions, visible moulds were noted in the wet samples, with *Penicillium*, *Eurotium* and *Aspergillus* comprising the predominant species.

Böhm and Hochleithner (1991) analysed exotic bird foods suspected of causing mycotoxicosis, and found that rearing food and millet seed cobs contained 20 and 15 ppb aflatoxin B_1 respectively. Loss of appetite, the appearance of neurological symptoms, and a high and rapid mortality in young birds formed the clinical symptoms of aflatoxicosis, and trichothecenes may exacerbate the symptoms. In an insect-infested food, trichothecenes (2 ppm nivalenol, 0.3 ppm deoxynivalenol and 0.1 ppm diacetoxyscirpenol) were identified by gas chromatography. Budgerigar food samples were found to be contaminated with *Mucor* spp. at a level of more than 1 million spores per gram. In all cases, changing to uncontaminated food was successful at reversing the clinical signs of mycotoxicosis.

Safe storage of pet food

All cans or bags of dog and cat food should be labelled with an appropriate shelf life. Expired food should not be used and opened cans or bags should be used within a reasonable amount of time to prevent spoilage by mould spores, insects, oxygen, moisture and UV light. Poorly stored pet food will oxidise, causing micronutrients and vitamins to degrade. Mouldy food will become contaminated with mycotoxins, and infestation of mites, bugs, and other storage pests use up the nutrients in the infested food. To limit the exposure of pet animals to mycotoxins, pet food should be purchased in amounts sufficient for one week, and the manufacturing date and shelf life of the product should be noted. Pet food should be kept in a cool dry environment, and larger bags can be stored in the freezer. Opened tins should be refrigerated. Always look at the sensory qualities of food before using it - never feed off-colours, rancid, mouldy, or off-flavoured food. If your pet suddenly doesn't want to eat the food, it should be discarded. Where owners are producing home-made food, always use fresh products and kept under appropriate conditions.

Manufacturers are not allowed to dilute a commodity containing excessive amounts of a mycotoxin (Dzanis, 2006). The issue of mycotoxins in raw ingredients is one of the most challenging for pet food manufacturers to successfully control. The very nature of mycotoxins makes them difficult to manage as each growing season is different and not every commodity is affected in the same way. Improper sampling and poor testing procedures can produce inaccurate results which can prove costly to rectify, if incorrect

(Maune, 2006). While aflatoxins, ochratoxins, and various *Fusarium* mycotoxins pose important health threats to dogs fed cereal-based dry diets, the application of new screening protocols, cereal processing techniques and dietary supplementation with mycotoxin-sequestering agents can offer solutions for the pet food industry (Leung and Smith, 2006a).

Conclusions

Problems associated with mycotoxin contamination are generally complex. *Aspergillus* spp., *Fusarium* spp., and *Penicillium* spp. can produce many different types of toxins, and contamination might occur anywhere in the production chain where cereals grains, soybean meal and their by-products feature. High temperature processing, such as extrusion or canning, cannot be relied upon to destroy mycotoxins, as these compounds are highly chemically stable, and very difficult to denature. Uncleaned grain (which retain their protective hull exterior) are more likely to be contaminated with fungus than cleaned grain. Aflatoxins, ochratoxins, cyclopiazonic acid, as well as fusariotoxins such as zearalenone, deoxynivalenol, moniliformin and fumonisins, are common, and all of them can be found in pet foods. Aflatoxins still dominate the list of high risk substances in pet foods. Contamination can occur directly through *A. flavus* infected cereal ingredients, or indirectly through residues in organs such as livers or kidneys from slaughtered animals, such as poultry, pigs or cattle that have been fed contaminated feed. Consequently, aflatoxicosis continues to be a problem and should be considered in a differential diagnosis for sick dogs. High aflatoxin contamination can be seen in peanuts or other kernels that are often the main ingredients of pet bird food.

As all mycotoxins affect animal health, they should be of concern to pet owners. Dose and time of oral ingestion affect the severity of the diseases. Usually toxicosis is associated with a combination of stress and exposure, giving rise to a variety of severe symptoms which, together, are classified as mycotoxicosis. Not unexpectedly, the symptoms of mycotoxicosis in pets are very similar to those seen in farm animals, and include jaundice, loss of appetite, and dizziness, and may cause severe organ changes including hepatitis, blood coagulation, neuronal symptoms, and even death in advanced cases.

Mycotoxins affect various organs and tissues, and combinations of fungal toxins (which are commonly found in naturally-infected raw materials) can be synergistic, leading to dramatic effects on animal health. One of the greatest concerns long-term, is the carcinogenicity associated with certain toxins (aflatoxins, fumonisins), as this has major implications for longer-lived companion species and their potential development of cancers. This aside, although acute mycotoxicosis rarely occurs, chronic cases are more common and can lead to increased susceptibility to infectious diseases, damage to the liver, kidney, and reproductive organs, poor coat condition, anorexia, food refusal, vomiting, and lethargy.

Fortunately, because strict quality control standards are practiced at pet food manufacturing plants (including screening of in-coming ingredients and cleaning of equipment) mycotoxin contamination of pet food is rare. Proper packaging and storage of feedstuffs has reduced the incidence of outbreaks associated with commercial food consumption. Application of mycotoxin-binding supplements can be added to ensure any toxins that have not been identified are inactivated, protecting the animal from potential harmful effects. The simplest precaution to prevent mycotoxicosis in pets is the avoidance of exposure to mould-spoiled foodstuffs, whether directly fed or within reach in their environment.

References

Armbrecht, B.H., Geleta, J.N., Shalkop, W.T. and Durbin, C.J. (1971). A sub-acute exposure of Beagle dogs to aflatoxin. *Toxicology and Applied Pharmacology* **18:** 579-585

Arp, L.H. and Richard, J.L. (1979). Intoxication of dogs with the mycotoxin penitrem A. *JAVMA* **175:** 565-566

Bailey, W.S. and Groth, A.H. (1959). The relationship of hepatitis X of dogs and mouldy corn poisoning of swine. *JAVMA* **134:** 514-516

Basalan, M., Hismiogullari, S.E., Hismiogullari, A.A., and Filazi, A. (2004). Fungi and aflatoxin B1 in horse and dog feeds in Western Turkey. *Revue Med Vet* **156 (5):** 248-252

Bastianello, S.S., Nesbit, J.W., Williams, M.C., and Lange, A.L. (1987). Pathological findings in a natural outbreak of aflatoxicosis in dogs. *Onderstepoort J Vet Res.* **54:** 635-640

Bingham, A.K., Huebner, H.J., Phillips, T.D. and Bauer, J.E. (2004). Identification and reduction of urinary aflatoxin metabolites in dogs. *Food and Chemical Toxicology* **42:** 1851-1858

Bingham, A.K., Phillips, T.D. and Bauer, J.E. (2003). Potential for dietary protection against the effects of aflatoxins in animals. *JAVMA* **222:** 591-595

Bird, C. (2000). Detecting and controlling mycotoxins in pet foods. *Technical Symposium on Mycotoxins.* Alltech Inc., Nicholasville, KY, USA.

Blank, R.; Höhler, D. and Wolffram S., (1999). Ochratoxin A in der Nahrungskette-Vorkommen Toxizität und Dekontamination. Übers. Tierernährung. **27:** 123-163

Böhm, J. (2000a). Fusariotoxins in animal nutrition. Habilitation Vetmed. Univ. Vienna

Böhm, J. (2000b). Fusariotoxins and their importance in animal nutrition. *Übers. Tierernährg.* **28**: 95-132.

Böhm, J. and Hochleithner, M. (1991). Mycotoxicosis in pet birds – selected cases. 1ˢᵗ Conference of the European Committee of the Association of Avian Veterinarians. Vienna, March 13-16. pp 255-257

Boysen, S.R., Rozanski, E.A., Chan, D.L., Grobe, T.L., Fallon, M.J. and Rush, J.E. (2002). Tremorgenic mycotoxicosis in four dogs from a single household. *JAVMA* **221**: 1441-1444

Bueno, D.J., Silva, J.O. and Oliver, G. (2001). Microflora in Commercial Pet Foods. *J Food Protection* **64**: 741-743

Canady, R. A., Coker, R. D., Egan, S. K., Krska, R., Kuiper-Goodman, Olsen, T. M., Pestka, J., Resnik S. and Schlatter J. (2002). The joint FAO/WHO expert committee on food additives (JECFA) Deoxynivalenol. http://www.inchem.org/documents/jecfa/jecmono/v47je05.htm, last access: 2003-12-9.

Coppock, RW, Hoffmann, WE, Gelberg, HB, Bass, D, Buck, WB. (1989). Haematological changes induced by intravenous administration of diacetoxyscirpenol in pigs, dogs, and calves. *Am J Vet Res.* **50**: 411-415.

Devegowda, G. (2000). Mycotoxins: hidden killers in pet foods. Is there a biological solution? In: *Technical Symposium on Mycotoxins*. Alltech Inc., Nicholasville KY

Edds, G.T. (1973). Acute aflatoxicosis: a review. *JAVMA* **162**: 304-309

Europäische Kommission (2003). Richtlinie 2003/100/EG der Kommission vom 31. Oktober 2003 zur Änderung von Anhang I zur Richtlinie 2002/32/EG des Europäischen Parlaments und des Rates über unerwünschte Stoffe in der Tierernährung; Abl. L 285 vom 1.11.2003, S. 33

Europäisches Schnellwarnsystem für Futtermittel (RASFF) (2006). Aflatoxins in feed for dogs 2006, Anl, 22.02.2006 (Information Notification)

Gareis, M., Reubel, G., Kröning, T. and Porzig, R. (1987). Ein Fall von infektiösem Welpensterben bei Afghanen in Verbindung mit der Verfütterung von Ochratoxin A – haltigem Milchpulver. *Tierärztl. Umschau* **42**: 77-80

Gareis, M. and Scheuer, R. (1999). Ochratoxin A in Fleisch und Fleischerzeugnissen. Proceedings 21. Mykotoxin-Workshop. p. 148

Greene, C.E., Barsanti, J.A. and Jones, B.D. (1977). Disseminated intravascular coagulation complicating aflatoxicosis in dogs. *Cornell Vet.* **67**: 29-49

Henke, S.E., Gallardo, V.C., Martinez, B. and Balley, R. (2001). Survey of aflatoxin concentrations in wild bird seed purchased in Texas. *J Wildl Dis.* **37:** 831-835

Hidy, PH., Baldwin, R.S., Greasham, R.L., Keith, C.L. and McMullen, J.R. (1977). Zearalenone and some derivates: Production and biological activities. In: *Adv. Appl. Microbiol.* (D. Perlman ed.) **22:** 59-82, Acad. Press, New York

Hocking, A.D., Holds, K., Tobin, N.F. (1988). Intoxication by tremorgenic mycotoxin (penitrem A) in a dog. *Aust Vet J.* **65:** 82-85

Hughes, D.M., Gahl, M.J., Graham, C.H. and Grieb S.L. (1999). Overt signs of toxicity to dogs and cats of dietary deoxynivalenol. *J. Anim. Sci.* **77:** 693-700

Hussein, S.H. and Brasel, J.M., (2001). Toxicity, metabolism, and impact of mycotoxins on humans and animals. *Toxicology* **167:** 101–134

Ketterer, P.J., Williams, E.S., Blaney, B.J. and Connole, M.D. (1975). Canine aflatoxicosis. *Aust Vet J.* **51:** 355- 357

Kitchen, D.N., Carlton, W.W. and Hinsman, E.J. (1977c). Ochratoxin A and citrinin induced nephrosis in Beagle dogs. III. Terminal renal ultra structural alterations. *Vet. Path.* **14:** 392-406

Kitchen, D.N., Carlton, W.W. and Tuite, J. (1977a). Ochratoxin A and citrinin induced nephrosis in Beagle dogs. I. Clinical and clinicopathological features. *Vet. Path.* **14:** 154- 172

Kitchen, D.N., Carlton, W.W. and Tuite, J. (1977b). Ochratoxin A and citrinin induced nephrosis in Beagle dogs. II. Pathology. *Vet Path.* **14:** 261-272

Kokkonen, M., Jestoi, M. and Rizzo, A. (2005). The effect of substrate on mycotoxin production of selected Penicillium strains. *Int J Food Microbiol.* **99:** 207-214

Krogh, P. (1992). Role of ochratoxin in disease causation. *Fd. Chem. Toxicol.* **30:** 213- 244

Liggett, A.D., Colvin, B.M., Beaver R.W. and Wilson, D.M. (1986). Canine Aflatoxicosis: A Continuing Problem. *Vet Hum Toxicol.* **28:** 428-430

Leung, M.C.K. and Smith, T. K. (2006a). Mycotoxin issues for dog food evaluated. *Feedstuffs*, July 31, 14-15

Leung, M.C.K. and Smith, T. K. (2006b). Effects of feeding a blend of grains naturally contaminated with Fusarium mycotoxins on feed intake and body weight of mature Beagle dogs. Poster presented at the Alltech's 22nd Annual Symposium.

Lutsky, I. and Mor, N. (1981). Experimental alimentary toxic aleukia in cats. *Lab Anim Sci.* **31:** 43-47

Maia, P.P., and Bastos de Sequeira, M.E.P. (2002). Occurrence of aflatoxins B1, B2, G1 and G2 in some Brazilian pet foods. *Food Additives and Contaminants* **19:** 1180-1183

Mellor, S. (2003). Keep petfood mycotoxins on the leash. *Feed Mix* **11:** 23-24

Mirocha, C.J., Christensen, C.M. and Nelson, G.H. (1968).

Physiologic activity of some fungal estrogens produced by Fusarium. *Cancer Res.* **28:** 2319-2322

Muirhead, S. (2006). Pet food varieties recalled. *Feedstuffs,* January 16, 2006, S. 3

Naude, T.W., O'Brien, O.M., Rundberget, T., McGregor, A.D., Roux, C. and Flaoyen, A. (2002). Tremorgenic neuromycotoxicosis in 2 dogs ascribed to the ingestion of penitrem A and possibly roquefortine in rice contaminated with Penicillium crustosum. *J S Afr Vet Assoc.* **73** (4): 211 – 215

Newberne, J.W., Bailey, W.S. and Seibold, H.R. (1955). Notes on a Recent Outbreak and Experimental Reproduction of Hepatitis in Dogs. *J. A.V.M.A.* **127:** 59-62

Newberne, P.M., Russo, R. and Wogan, G.N. (1966). Acute Toxicity of Aflatoxin B1 in the Dog. *Path. Vet.* **3:** 331-340

Nuehring, L.P., Rowland, G.N., Harrison, L.R., Cole, R.J. and Dorner, J.W. (1985). Cyclopiazonic acid mycotoxicosis in the dog. *Am J Vet Res* **46:** 1670-1676

Patterson, D.S.P. (1977). Toxin-producing fungi and susceptible animal species. In: Wyllie and Morehouse, Mycotoxic Fungi, Mycotoxins, Mycotoxicosis Vol.1, Marcel Dekker Inc. pp. 156-158

Pier, A.C., Richard, J.L. and Cysewski, S.J. (1980). Implications of mycotoxins in animal disease. *JAVMA* **176:** 719-724

Pühringer, S. (2003): Untersuchungen zum Vorkommen von Ochratoxin A in Katzennieren und Katzenfuttermitteln. Diss. Vetmed. Univ. Wien

Puls, R. and Ladyman, E. (1988) : Roquefortine toxicity in a dog. *Can Vet J.* **29:** 569

Puschner. B. (2002). Mycotoxins. *Vet Clin Small Anim* **32:** 409-419

Razzazi-Fazeli, E., Böhm, J., Grajewski, J., Szczepaniak, K., Kübber-Heiss, A. and Iben, C. (2001). Residues of ochratoxin A in pet foods, canine and feline kidneys. *J Anim Physiol a. Anim Nutr* **85:** 212-216

Razzazi-Fazeli, E., Böhm, J., Adler, A. and Zentek, J. (2003). Fusarientoxine und ihre Bedeutung in der Nutztierfütterung, eine Übersicht. *Wiener Tierärztliche Monatsschrift* **90:** 202-210

Rumbeiha, W.K. (2000): Clinical implications of mycotoxicosis in companion animals, Technical Symposium on Mycotoxins. Nicholasville, KY. 10-3-2000

Rumbeiha, W. (2003). Mycotoxicosis in pets, rare but ruthless. *Feed Tech* **7(3):** 25-27

Schell, M.M. (2000). Tremorgenic mycotoxin intoxication. "Toxicology brief" in issue April, *Vet Med*

Scudamore, K.A, (2005) Principles and applications of mycotoxin analysis In: *The Mycotoxin Blue Book* ed. D Diaz. Nottingham

University Press, Nottingham, UK.

Scudamore, K.A., Hetmanski, M.T., Nawaz, S., Naylor, J. and Rainbird, S. (1997). Determination of mycotoxins in pet foods sold for domestic pets and wild birds using linked-column immunoassay clean-up and HPLC. *Food Additives and Contaminants*, **14:** 175-186

Seibold, H.R. (1953). Hepatitis X in dogs. *Vet Med.* **48:** 242-243

Seibold, H.R. and Bailey, W.S. (1952): An epizootic of hepatitis in dogs. *JAVMA* **121:** 201-206

Sharma, M. and Marquez, C. (2001). Determination of aflatoxins in domestic pet foods (dog and cat) using immunoaffinity column and HPLC. *Anim. Feed Science and Technology* **93:** 109-114

Smith, A.J., Stenske, K.A., Bartges, J.W. and Kirk, C.A. (2005). Diet-associated hepatic failure and immune-mediated hemolytic anemia in a Weimaraner. *J Vet Emerg Crit Care* **16:** 42-47

Songsermsakul, P., Razzazi, E., Böhm, J. and Zentek, J. (2004). Occurrence of deoxynivalenol (DON) and ochratoxin (OTA) in dog foods. 26. Mykotoxin-Workshop, 17.-19. Mai 2004, Herrsching am Ammersee, S. 95

Stenske, K.A., Smith, J.R., Newman, S.J., Newman, L.B. and Kirk, C.A. (2006). Aflatoxicosis in dogs and dealing with suspected contaminated commercial foods. *JAVMA* **228:** 1686-91

Szczech, G.M., Carlton, W.W. and Hinsman, E.J. (1974). Ochratoxicosis in Beagle dogs. III. Terminal renal ultrastructural alterations. *Vet. Path.* **11:** 385-406

Szczech, G.M., Carlton, W.W. and Tuite, J. (1973a) Ochratoxicosis in Beagle dogs. I. Clinical and clinicopathological features. *Vet. Path.* **10:** 135-154

Szczech, G.M., Carlton, W.W. and Tuite, J. (1973b). Ochratoxicosis in Beagle dogs. II. Pathology. *Vet. Path.* **10:** 219-231

Statist. Zentralamt (2001): ftp://www.statistik.at/pub/neuerscheinungen/freizeit2001.pdf

Water, S.L. (2002). Acute penitrem A and roquefortine poisoning in a dog. *Can Vet J.* **43 (5):** 372 - 374

Wolf-Hall, C.E., Hanna, M.A. and Bullerman, L.B. (1999). Stability of deoxynivalenol in heat-treated foods. *J Food Prot.* **62:** 962-964

Wolter, R. and Jean, C. (1997) Intoxications alimentaires: principales mycotoxicoses chez les carnivores domestiques. *Prat Med Chir Anim Comp* **32:** 157-162

Young, K.L., Villar, D., Carson, T.L., Ierman, P.M., Moore, R.A. and Bottoff, M.R. (2003). Tremorgenic mycotoxin intoxication with penitrem A and roquefortine in two dogs. *JAVMA* **222:** 52-53

Zwierzchovski, W., Gajecki, M., Obremski, K., Zielonka, L., and Baranowski, M. (2004). The occurrence of zearalenone and its derivates in standard and therapeutic feeds for companion animals. *Pol J Vet Sci* **7(4):** 289-293

Exploiting molecular biology for pet health and disease research: brain aging

Kelly S. Swanson

Brain health of aging dogs

Over the past few decades, canine life span has continued to increase, due in part to improved veterinary care, vaccination programs, and nutritional status. It is estimated that one third to one half of today's pet dogs and cats are considered to be "senior" (> 7 years of age) (Lund et al., 1999). Similar to humans, geriatric dogs have an increased incidence of medical complications and complex diseases. One age-related disease receiving considerable attention in recent years is that of cognitive dysfunction. Canine Cognitive Dysfunction Syndrome (CDS) has been proposed to describe the progressive neurodegenerative disorder of senior dogs (Ruehl et al., 1995). Dogs with CDS may display several abnormal behaviors including spatial disorientation and/or confusion, altered learning and memory, activity changes (purposeless, repetitive, or decreased), altered social relationships, altered sleep-wake cycles, increased anxiety or restlessness, altered appetite and/or self-hygiene, and decreased perception and/or responsiveness (Landsberg and Araujo, 2005). Although the age of onset may be 11 years old or greater before clinical signs become apparent to owners, recent findings suggest that cognitive decline can be detected as early as 6 years of age in a laboratory environment (Araujo, 2004).

General physiologic changes associated with aging tissues include progressive organ degeneration (lack of reserve), tissue hypoxia, decreased enzyme systems, behavioral changes, dryness of mucosal tissues, cellular membrane alterations, and decreased immune surveillance (Fortney, 2001). Many of these age-related changes are thought to contribute to the development of disease. With age, numerous anatomic changes occur within brain tissue, including decreased brain mass, increased ventricular size, meningeal calcification, demyelination, and glial changes (increased size and number of astrocytes), increased lipofuscin concentration, increased number of apoptic bodies, neuroaxonal degeneration, and a decreased number of neurons (Su et al., 1998; Borras et al., 1999). Functional changes such as decreased catecholamine neurotransmitters, increased monoamine oxidase B activity, and decreased cholinergic activity also occur with age (Milgram et al., 1993; Gerlach et al., 1994). ß-amyloid deposition is virtually undetectable in young dogs, but can be extensive in the elderly (Cummings et al., 1996).

Similar to humans, ß-amyloid deposition is strongly associated with cognitive dysfunction (increased error rate in discriminatory, reversal and spatial learning tests) in dogs (Head et al., 1998). In addition to ß-amyloid, several proteins are known to contribute to the pathology of neurodegenerative diseases including normal tau protein, synaptic proteins, amyloid precursor protein (APP), and apolipoprotein E (APOE). Although strong correlations exist between these proteins and cognitive dysfunction, few mechanisms by which they contribute to disease have been demonstrated.

Oxidative stress is known to contribute to genomic instability and cellular senescence, and thus, is one of the most popular theories of aging (Finkel and Holbrook, 2000). Reactive oxygen species such as superoxide anion, hydrogen peroxide, and hydroxyl radicals are generated by metabolism and cause molecular damage to proteins, lipids, and nucleic acids. Because mitochondria are the major site of free radical production, they are often the primary target for oxidative damage and subsequent dysfunction. Researchers have demonstrated that as mitochondria age, they become less efficient and produce a greater amount of free radicals and less energy compared to younger mitochondria (Shigenaga et al., 1994).

Postmitotic cells are thought to be the most susceptible to oxidative damage because of their inability to replace themselves. Therefore, organs such as the brain, heart, and skeletal muscle may be the most vulnerable to oxidative damage. Anderson et al. (2000) demonstrated a correlation between DNA damage, much of which is caused by oxidative damage, and amyloid ß-peptide (Aß) deposition in brain tissue of aged dogs. In vitro, Aß has been shown to trigger degeneration of cultured neurons through activation of an apoptotic pathway (Loo et al., 1993). Although apoptotic cell number and ß-amyloid plaques have not been significantly correlated in all experiments, the correlation between apoptotic cell number and dementia index was significant in the study reported by Kiatipattanasakul et al. (1996). Thus, while it appears that both DNA damage and ß-amyloid deposition are associated with cognitive dysfunction, it is unclear whether these events act in concert or are independent of one another.

Current dietary intervention strategies

Due to the evidence of oxidative damage and its impact on aging tissues, many dietary strategies involve the body's natural antioxidant defense systems, altering enzymes such as superoxide dismutase, catalase, and glutathione peroxidase or supplementing free radical scavengers such as vitamins A, C, and E. For example, an antioxidant-rich diet supplemented with vitamins E and C, ß-carotene, selenium, DL-α-lipoic acid, L-carnitine, and various other flavonoids and carotenoids contained in spinach flakes, tomato pomace, grape pomace, carrot granules, and citrus pulp, has been reported to improve cognitive performance in aged dogs (Siwak et al., 2005).

Dietary fat and cholesterol inclusion levels and fatty acid form may also impact cognitive development and the effects of aging on brain health. It has been reported that both the generation and clearance of Aß are regulated by cholesterol, which modulates the processing of both APP and Aß. Elevated cholesterol level increases Aß in cellular and most animal models and is a risk factor for Alzheimer's disease (Jarvik et al., 1995). Dietary fat intake has also been associated with psychosocial and cognitive function in young children. While total fat and saturated fat intake were unrelated to performance on achievement and intelligence tests, cholesterol and polyunsaturated fatty acid intakes were associated with decreased and increased performance, respectively (Zhang et al., 2005). Supplementation of a *Ginkgo biloba* extract is believed to improve cognitive function in Alzheimer's disease patients, possibly by inhibiting ß-amyloid production by lowering free cholesterol levels as demonstrated in aged rats (Yao et al., 2004).

A specific group of lipids, the omega-3 fatty acids, have been tested for their beneficial effects on brain health. Whalley et al. (2004) reported improved cognition in elderly humans consuming food supplements containing omega-3 fatty acids and having greater erythrocyte omega-3 fatty acid concentrations. Docosahexaenoic acid (DHA; 22:6n-3), a product of the omega-3 pathway, appears to play an important role in neuronal development and cognitive function. Kelley (2005) reported that a diet containing elevated concentrations of omega-3 fatty acids (including DHA) resulted in greater erythrocyte DHA concentrations in pregnant bitches throughout gestation, greater erythrocyte DHA concentrations in offspring, and increased trainability of offspring, substantiating the importance of this fatty acid in the neurological development of dogs.

Using genomic biology to study brain health

While numerous anatomic changes to brain tissue have been associated with aging, very few exact mechanisms responsible for these changes and their impact on cognitive function have been identified. Besides the inaccessibility to brain tissue, limiting factors include the complexity of brain function, the numerous genetic and environmental factors contributing to brain health, and the time and costs associated with executing these experiments. In addition to improved imaging technologies that enable researchers to scan brain tissue in vivo, recent advances in genomic biology have greatly expanded research opportunities. Applying genomic tools and concepts to companion animal research will greatly enhance our understanding of the aging process and its impact on brain health.

Efforts put forth by the National Institutes of Health (NIH) have resulted in genome sequencing of numerous animal models, including the dog and cat. Based on sequence data generated by recent canine sequencing projects (Kirkness et al., 2003; Lindblad-Toh et al., 2005), a canine SNP (single nucleotide polymorphism) map is also being developed (www.genome.gov/12511476). Canine genome sequence data enables genome scanning experiments to be performed. These experiments may be critical in the study of canine aging by identifying genetic loci or gene clusters contributing to age-related diseases. Human experiments have already identified associations between genetic polymorphisms present in the APOE gene and brain health. A recent study identified the APOE e4 allele as a strong risk factor for increased amyloid deposition and cognitive impairment in humans (Bennett et al., 2005). Human studies have also identified correlations between interleukin-1 (IL-1) variants having increased levels of inflammatory mediators and increased severity of several chronic diseases, including Alzheimer's disease (Griffin et al., 2000; Grimaldi et al., 2000). SNP assessment in dogs may identify genetic profiles associated with age-related disease incidence in dogs, including those associated with brain health.

In addition to the availability of canine genome sequence data, tools used to measure mRNA and protein concentrations continue to be developed and improved. Current techniques not only have a much lower detection limit than previous methods, but are more accurate and can be automated. Moreover, "high-throughput" techniques such as DNA microarrays enable the measurement of thousands of mRNA transcripts simultaneously, providing researchers with a holistic view of a cell, tissue, or organism. Microarray analysis is a popular strategy used to identify genes and biological pathways associated with complex diseases that are poorly understood. Genes significantly up- or down-regulated in the diseased state can then be studied in more detail in subsequent experiments.

DNA microarrays have been used to study aged brain tissue of mice (Lee et al., 2000; Jiang et al., 2001; Weindruch et al., 2002), humans (Lu et al., 2004), and dogs (Swanson et al., 2006). In general, aging seems to result in a gene expression profile indicative of an inflammatory response, oxidative stress, and reduced neurotrophic support (Lee et al., 2000; Lu et al., 2004). Moreover, genes associated with protein turnover and growth and trophic factors were decreased in aged mice (Lee et al., 2000), while those playing a role in synaptic function and plasticity that underlies learning and memory were among those most significantly affected in aged human brain tissue (Lu et al., 2004). Jiang et al. (2001) also noted that proteases that play an essential role in regulating neuropeptide metabolism, APP processing, and neuronal apoptosis were upregulated in aged brain, suggesting a major role in brain aging. We observed similar results in aged dog brain tissues, with genes associated with inflammatory response and oxidative stress having increased expression. Interestingly, two peptides shown to increase cognitive performance, somatostatin and neuropeptide Y, had decreased expression levels in aged dogs (Swanson et al., 2006).

While DNA microarrays have had a major positive impact on biological research, they do have limitations. Besides the semi-quantitative nature of microarrays that requires validation by quantitative reverse-transcriptase polymerase chain reaction (qRT-PCR), a low correlation between protein and mRNA concentration is observed for some genes. Discrepancies may be due to a number of factors, including the level at which a gene is regulated (e.g., transcription vs. translation) and the occurrence of post-translational modifications. Thus, a great need for techniques able to identify and quantify proteins exists. Experiments using proteomic analysis to evaluate aged brain tissues in rodent models have recently been reported (Poon et al., 2005). These preliminary experiments substantiate the oxidative damage theory of aging, as increased concentrations of oxidized proteins were detected in many of these aged tissues. More of these efforts are required to complement the mRNA datasets being generated, measure post-translational modifications of newly synthesized proteins, and detect the amount and type of protein damage in tissues of aged animals.

Conclusions

Canine Cognitive Dysfunction Syndrome (CDS) is common in the elderly dog population. Dogs with CDS share many of the same anatomical characteristics (e.g., amyloid deposition) as human Alzheimer's patients. While it is well known that many of these anatomical changes are highly correlated with cognition, the factors responsible for these changes are largely unknown in both species. Some researchers have reported increased cognitive performance by supplementing natural antioxidants, omega-3 fatty acid treatments, or herbal remedies. However, the mechanisms by which these nutrients function are not entirely understood. Given the recent availability of canine genome sequence data and powerful molecular biological tools, it is now possible to identify genes and biological pathways involved with neurological pathologies such as CDS. Incorporating these datasets and techniques into this field of research is critical, as scientists may soon identify genotypes most susceptible to disease, develop dietary strategies that prevent or prolong the development of cognitive decline, or develop effective pharmaceutical therapeutics.

References

Anderson, A. J., W. W. Ruehl, L. K. Fleischmann, K. Stenstrom, T. L. Entriken, and B. J. Cummings. (2000). DNA damage and apoptosis in the aged canine brain: Relationship to Aß deposition in the absence of neuritic pathology. *Prog. Neuro-Psychopharmacol. Biol. Psychiat.* **24**: 787-799.

Araujo, J. A. (2004). Age-dependent learning and memory decline in dogs: Assessment and effectiveness of various interventions. *Presented at the 141ˢᵗ American Veterinary Medical Association Conference, Schaumberg, IL.*

Bennett, D. A., J. A. Schneider, R. S. Wilson, J. L. Bienias, E. Berry-Kravis, and S. E. Arnold. (2005). Amyloid mediates the association of apolipoprotein E e4 allele to cognitive function in older people. *J. Neurol. Neurosurg. Psychiatry* **76**: 1194-1199.

Borras, D., I. Ferrer, and M. Pumarola. (1999). Age related changes in the brain of the dog. *Vet. Pathol.* **36**: 202-211.

Cummings, B. J., E. Head, A. J. Afagh, N. W. Milgram, and C. W. Cotman. (1996). ß-amyloid accumulation correlates with cognitive dysfunction in the aged canine. *Neurobiol. Learning Memory* **66**: 11-23.

Finkel, T., and N. Holbrook. (2000). Oxidants, oxidative stress and the biology of ageing. *Nature* **408**: 239-247.

Fortney, W. D. (2001). Clinical perspectives and issues related to senior companion animals. Proceedings from a Pre-Congress Symposium: *World Small Animal Veterinary Association, World Congress 2001. The Iams Company, Dayton, OH.*

Gerlach, M., P. Riederer, and M. B. H. Youdim. (1994). Effects of disease and aging on monoamine oxidases A and B. Pages 21-30 in *Monoamine Oxidase Inhibitors in Neurological Diseases* (Lieberman, A., C. W. Olanow, and M. B. H. Youdim, eds). Marcel Dekker, New York, NY.

Griffin W. S., J. A. Nicoll, L. M. Grimaldi, J. G. Sheng, and R. E. Mrak. (2000). The pervasiveness of interleukin-1 in Alzheimer pathogenesis: A role for specific polymorphisms in disease risk. *Exp. Gerontol.* **35**: 481-487.

Grimaldi L. M., V. M. Casadei, C. Ferri, F. Veglia, F. Licastro, G. Annoni, I. Biunno, G. De Bellis, S. Sorbi, C. Mariani, N. Canal, W. S. Griffin, and M. Franceschi. (2000). Association of early-onset Alzheimer's disease with an interleukin-1 alpha gene polymorphism. *Ann. Neurol.* **47**: 361-365.

Head, E., H. Callahan, B. A. Muggenburg, C. W. Cotman, and N. W. Milgram. (1998). Visual-discrimination learning ability and beta-amyloid accumulation in the dog. *Neurobiol. Aging* **19**: 415-425.

Jarvik, G. P., E. M. Wijsman, W. A. Kukull, G. D. Schellenberg, C. Yu, and E. B. Larson. (1995). Interactions of apolipoprotein E genotype, total cholesterol level, age, and sex in prediction of Alzheimer's disease: a case-control study. *Neurol.* **45**: 1092-1096.

Jiang, C. H., J. Z. Tsien, P. G. Schultz, and Y. Hu. (2001). The effects of aging on gene expression in the hypothalamus and cortex of mice. *Proc. Natl. Acad. Sci.* **98**: 1930-1934.

Kelley, R. (2005). Improving puppy trainability through nutrition. Pages 11-15 in *Proceedings from Symposium: Federation of Animal Science Societies FASS 2005 Joint Annual Meeting. The Iams Company, Dayton, OH.*

Kiatipattanasakul, W., S.-I. Nakamura, M. M. Hossain, H. Nakayama, T. Uchino, S. Shumiya, N. Goto, and K. Doi. (1996). Apoptosis in the aged dog brain. *Acta Neuropathol.* **92**: 242-248.

Kirkness E. F., V. Bafna, A. L. Halpern, S. Levy, K. Remington, D. B. Rusch, A. L. Delcher, M. Pop, W. Wang, C. M. Fraser, and J. C. Venter. (2003). The dog genome: Survey sequencing and comparative analysis. *Science* **301**: 1898-1903.

Landsberg, G., and J. A. Araujo. (2005). Behavior problems in geriatric pets. *Vet. Clin. Small Anim.* **35**: 675-698.

Lee, C.-K., R. Weindruch, and T. A. Prolla. (2000). Gene-expression profile of the ageing brain in mice. *Nature Genet.* **25**: 294-297.

Lindblad-Toh, K., C. M. Wade, T. S. Mikkelsen, et al. (2005). Genome sequence, comparative analysis and haplotypes structure of the domestic dog. *Nature* **438**: 803-819.

Loo, D. T., A. Copani, C. J. Pike, E. R. Whittemore, A. J. Walencewicz, and C. W. Cotman. (1993). Apoptosis is induced by ß-amyloid in cultured central nervous system neurons.

Proc. Natl. Acad. Sci. **90**: 7951-7955.

Lund, E. M., P. J. Armstrong, C. A. Kirk, L. M. Kolar, and J. S. Klausner. (1999). Health status and population characteristics of dogs and cats examined at private veterinary practices in the United States. *J. Am. Vet. Med. Assoc.* **214**: 1336-1341.

Lu, T., Y. Pan, S.-Y. Kao, C. Li, I. Kohane, J. Chan, and B. A. Yankner. (2004). Gene regulation and DNA damage in the ageing human brain. *Nature* **429**: 883-891.

Milgram, N. W., G. O. Ivy, E. Head, M. P. Murphy, P. H. Wu, W. W. Ruehl, P. H. Yu, D. A. Durden, B. A. Davis, I. A. Paterson, and A. A. Boulton. (1993). The effect of L-deprenyl on behavior, cognitive function, and biogenic amines in the dog. *Neurochem. Res.* **18**: 1211-1219.

Poon, H. F., R. A. Vaishnav, T. V. Getchell, M. L. Getchell, and D. A. Butterfield. (2005). Quantitative proteomics analysis of differential protein expression and oxidative modification of specific proteins in the brains of old mice. *Neurobiol. Aging (in press)*.

Ruehl, W. W., D. S. Bruyette, A. DePaoli, C. W. Cotman, E. Head, N. W. Milgram, and B. Cummings. (1995). Canine cognitive dysfunction as a model for human age-related cognitive decline, dementia and Alzheimer's disease: clinical presentation, cognitive testing, pathology and response to L-deprenyl therapy. *Prog. Brain Res.* **106**: 217-225.

Shigenaga, M. K., T. M. Hagen, and B. N. Ames. (1994). Oxidative damage and mitochondrial decay in aging. *Proc. Natl. Acad. Sci.* **91**: 10771-10778.

Siwak, C. T., P. D. Tapp, E. Head, S. C. Zicker, H. L. Murphey, B. A. Muggenburg, C. J. Ikeda-Douglas, C. W. Cotman, and N. W. Milgram. (2005). *Prog. Neuro-Psychopharmacol. Biol. Psychiat.* **29**: 461-469.

Su, M. Y., E. Head, W. M. Brooks, Z. Wang, B. A. Muggenburg, G. E. Adam, R. Sutherland, C. W. Cotman, and O. Nalcioglu. (1998). Magnetic resonance imaging of anatomic and vascular characteristics in a canine model of human aging. *Neurobiol. Aging* **19**: 479-485.

Swanson, K. S., C. J. Apanavicius, B. M. Vester, and N. A. Kirby. (2006). Impact of age on gene expression profiles of canine brain tissue. 2006 *J. Anim. Sci.* **84** (Suppl. 1): 172.

Weindruch, R., T. Kayo, C.-K. Lee, and T. A. Prolla. (2002). Gene expression profiling of aging using DNA microarrays. *Mech. Ageing Dev.* **123**: 177-193.

Whalley, L. J., H. C. Fox, K. W. Wahle, J. M. Starr, and I. J. Deary. (2004). Cognitive aging, childhood intelligence, and the use of food supplements: possible involvement of n-3 fatty acids. *Am. J. Clin. Nutr.* **80**: 1650-1657.

Yao, Z.-X., Z. Han, K. Drieu, and V. Papadopoulos. (2004). *Ginkgo biloba* extract (Egb 761) inhibits ß-amyloid production by lowering free cholesterol levels. *J. Nutr. Biochem.* **15**: 749-756.

Zhang, J., J. R. Hebert, and M. F. Muldoon. (2005). Dietary fat intake is associated with psychosocial and cognitive functioning of school-aged children in the United States. *J. Nutr.* **135**: 1967-1973.